Preface

Anatomy is in the crossroads of technological advancement. Human anatomy changes slowly but the technological options for teaching human anatomy change very quickly. The last decade has seen a revolution in the digital resources available to students and faculty. Computers and blackboard based instruction become more important to teaching and learning. New methods and innovations are changing the learning outcome, attitude and skill about the subject matter. The big volume anatomy books are getting support from the maneuverable up-to-date component manuals. A student completes one region of anatomy at a time. It is more comfortable for a student to carry that particular regional anatomy for the particular period of time. Anatomy is a visual science; it is much easier to imagine structures and grasp functional concepts through short description with clinical relevance. Currently, almost every student has a computer along with internet access and a student can easily visualize a life picture and get information. The purpose of this book is to provide book a significant guide to a novice student, refresher, and clinicians. "Upper Limb Anatomy Tutor" reflects my over nineteen years of teaching experience in three continents in different types of learning institutes.

This book is succinctly written in summary format. However, it is clear, complete and easily readable. The general organization of this book is to help an average student to be successful in the course and board examinations. All the essential parts of anatomy such as osteology, radiological anatomy, surface anatomy, along with a number of tables are added in this book to present all the information in a handy manner. Multiple groups of objective and viva voce questions are added to keep students prepared properly. I am eager to get feedback from my students and from my colleagues. Clinical correlations, clinical questions and case studies have been included to motivate the students and to make them aware of the applications and importance of basic anatomy to clinical science. This book is a useful tool to correlate the anatomical knowledge to the case scenario that a physician or a therapist may face on a daily basis.

I would like to acknowledge all individuals who were involved in the completion of this book. I particularly give heartfelt and sincere thanks to my wife Dr. Sultana for her love, patience and support, which has sustained me, making the completion of this book possible. My only son D.M. Suja helped me in computer set ups for the tables and figures.

I am deeply indebted to Dr. Shawn He M.D., M.S., for checking spelling, stylistic, and factual mistakes. His kind involvement has inspired me. It was a privilege to present my manuscript to a highly esteemed colleague.

I admit that there might be errors within the book in spite of repeated proof reading. Any suggestions to improve the book are encouraged and appreciated. Please send your suggestions via e-mail at dewanraja@hotmail.com

Sincerely,

Dewan S. Raja MBBS,MPhil,MPH,CPH,CHES,DTM&TH

Table of contents

Introduction   1
Osteology and Radiology of Upper limb   2
Scapula   3
Clavicle   9
Joints of the pectoral region   14
Humerus   19
Radius and Ulna   29
Elbow joint   31
Carpal Bones   37
Joints of the wrist, hand, and fingers   41
X-Ray of the wrist and hand   45
Shoulder and scapular region   47
Muscles of the scapular region   54
Quadrangular and triangular spaces   59
Triangular space and Triangular interval   60
Axillary nerve   61
Anastomosis around the scapula   62
 Arm   63
Muscles of the arm   65
Transverse section of the arm   69
Brachial artery   70
Anastomosis around the elbow joint   71
Radial nerve in the arm   72
Musculocutaneous nerve in the arm   73
Median nerve and Ulnar nerve in the arm   74
 Cubital fossa   75
Axilla   78
Muscles of the axilla   83
Brachial plexus   85
Important veins of the upper limb   93
Forearm   96

Flexor muscles of the
forearm   96
Back of the forearm   102
Radial nerve in the forearm   104
Ulnar nerve in the forearm   105
Deep muscles of the back of the forearm   106
Dorsum and Palm of the hand   109
Anatomical snuff box   109
Extensor retinaculum of the wrist   110
Flexor retinaculum   116
Vessels , nerves, and muscles of the hand   120
Palmer aponeurosis   124
Intrinsic muscles of the hand   127
Cutaneous nerves of the upper limb   140
Lymphatic system of the upper limb   143

Table of contents

Introduction   1

Osteology and Radiology of Upper limb   2

Scapula   3

Clavicle   9

Joints of the pectoral region   14

Humerus   19

Radius and Ulna   29

Elbow joint   31

Carpal Bones   37

Joints of the wrist, hand, and fingers   41

X-Ray of the wrist and hand   45

Shoulder and scapular region   47

Muscles of the scapular region   54

Quadrangular and triangular spaces   59

Triangular space and Triangular interval   60

Axillary nerve   61

Anastomosis around the scapula   62

Arm   63

Muscles of the arm   65

Transverse section of the arm   69

Brachial artery   70

Anastomosis around the elbow joint   71

Radial nerve in the arm   72

Musculocutaneous nerve in the arm   73

Median nerve and Ulnar nerve in the arm   74

Cubital fossa   75

Axilla   78

Muscles of the axilla   83

Brachial plexus   85

Important veins of the upper limb   93

Forearm   96

Flexor muscles of the
forearm   96
Back of the forearm   102
Radial nerve in the forearm   104
Ulnar nerve in the forearm   105
Deep muscles of the back of the forearm   106
Dorsum and Palm of the hand   109
Anatomical snuff box   109
Extensor retinaculum of the wrist   110
Flexor retinaculum   116
Vessels , nerves, and muscles of the hand   120
Palmer aponeurosis   124
Intrinsic muscles of the hand   127
Cutaneous nerves of the upper limb   140
Lymphatic system of the upper limb   143

Upper Limb Anatomy Tutor

The upper limb is made up of four regions: 1. shoulder; 2. brachium or arm 3.antebrachium or forearm; and 4. Manus or hand.

The shoulder region includes: a. the pectoral region including the breast; b. the axilla or armpit; and c. the scapular region. The bones of the shoulder region are the clavicle and the scapula. The clavicle articulates with the axial skeleton at the sternoclavicular joint while the scapula does not. The scapula is held in position by muscles. The clavicle articulates with the scapula at the acromioclavicular joint.

The arm extends from the shoulder joint to the elbow joint. The bone of the arm is the humerus. The humerus articulates with the scapula above and radius and ulna below.

The forearm extends from the elbow joint to the wrist joint. The bones of the forearm are the radius and the ulna. The radius and ulna articulates above with the humerus to form the elbow joint. They articulate with the carpal bones below to form the wrist joint. The radius and ulna meet each other to form the superior, middle and inferior radioulnar joints. An interosseous membrane attaches the interosseous borders of the radius and ulna along their shafts.

The hand includes: a. the wrist, supported by eight carpal bones arranged in two rows; b. the hand proper, supported by five metacarpal bones; and c. five digits(thumb, index finger, middle finger, ring finger, and little fingers). Each finger is supported by three phalanges, but the thumb has only two phalanges. There are 14 phalanges in total.

The upper and lower limbs were developed mainly for bearing the weight of the body and for locomotion. Nonetheless, with the evolution of the erect posture in human, the role of weight-bearing was taken over by the lower limbs. The upper limb has multiple movements in a series of joints. The human hand is a grasping device adaptable to perform various precise functions. Mankind is the master of the world because of the skilled movements of the hand.

Osteology and Radiology of the Upper Limb

X-Ray of the shoulder joint: Basic views include External and Internal Rotation. The "Scapular Y" view is an additional view to evaluate shoulder dislocations. (Wikipedia.org; Free Encyclopedia)

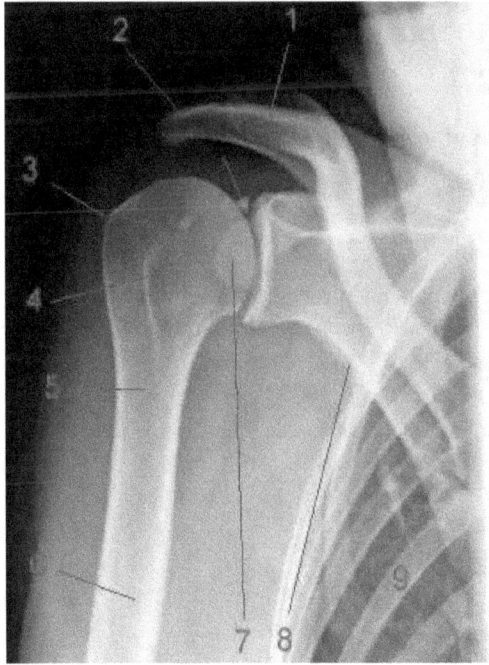

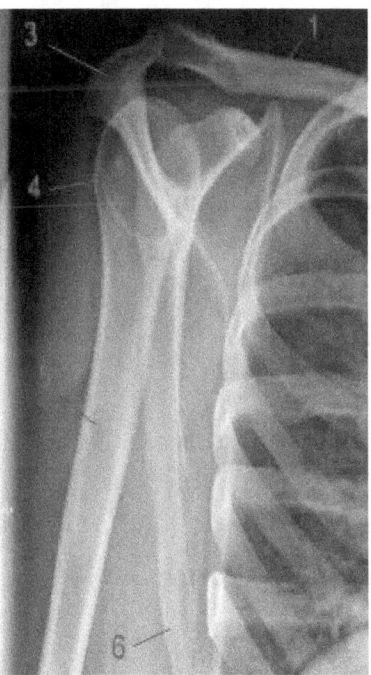

Shoulder X-Ray: Anteroposterior view

Shoulder X-Ray: Lateral view

1.	Clavicle
2.	Acromion
3.	Greater tubercle
4.	Lesser tubercle
5.	Neck of Humerus
6.	Humerus
7.	Coracoid Process
8.	Axillary border of scapula
9.	Rib

1.	Coracoid Process
2.	Clavicle
3.	Acromion
4.	Head of Humerus
5.	Humerus
6.	Axillary border of scapula

The scapula

The scapula is a **flat** bone lying against the posterior aspect of the rib cage. It has a **palpable** spine, acromion process, coracoid process, vertebral border, and an inferior angle. **The scapula is surrounded by muscles and seldom fractures.**

Anatomical position and side determination of the scapula

The scapula should be held by the same hand to which side it belongs.

1. The costal surface is directed forward and medially.

2. The glenoid cavity faces laterally with slightly forward and upward tilt.

3. The tip of the coracoid process is directed almost straight forward.

Coracoid Process of the Scapula

It is a curved bony process from the upper part of the head of the scapula.

Muscular Attachments of the Coracoid Process

Origin of—1. Short head of biceps brachii 2. Coracobrachialis

These two muscles take origin from the tip of the coracoid process by a common tendon. The coracobrachialis lies medially and the short head of biceps brachii lies laterally.

The pectoralis minor **inserts** on the medial border and superior surface of the coracoid process of the scapula.

Attachment of Ligaments to the Coracoid Process

1. Coracoclavicular ligament 2.Coracoacromial ligament and 3.Coraco-humeral ligament

The coracoacromial ligament passes on tensile force from the coracoid process to the acromion process and spine of the scapula.

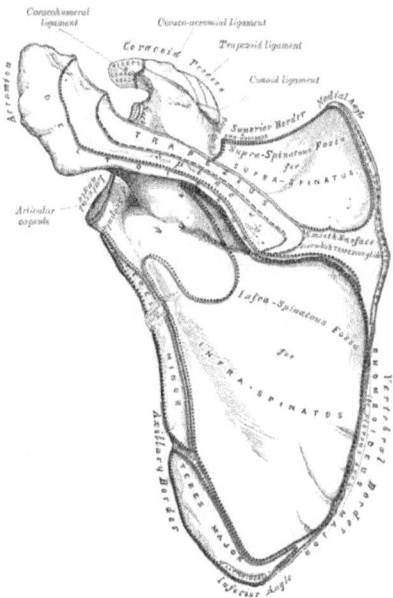

(Wikipedia.org; Free Encyclopedia)

Acromion Process of the Scapula

The acromion process continues from the lateral end of the spine of the scapula and it projects forwards to hang over the glenoid cavity. The acromion process has lateral and medial borders. It is subcutaneous throughout its course. The medial border has a small oval facet for articulation with the lateral end of the clavicle forming the acromioclavicular joint. The **acromioclavicular joint is a plane type of synovial joint.**

Muscular attachments of the acromion process

1. Deltoid muscle—originates from the lateral border of the acromion process

2. Trapezius muscle---inserts to the medial border of the acromion process

Attachment of Ligaments to the Acromion Process

1. Coracoacromial ligament and 2. Articular capsule of the acromioclavicular joint

Notes: The **scapula is entrenched in muscles** and rarely fractured. The spine and acromion process are palpable along their lengths. The inferior angle and medial margin can also be easily palpated through the skin.
(Wikipedia.org; Free Encyclopedia)

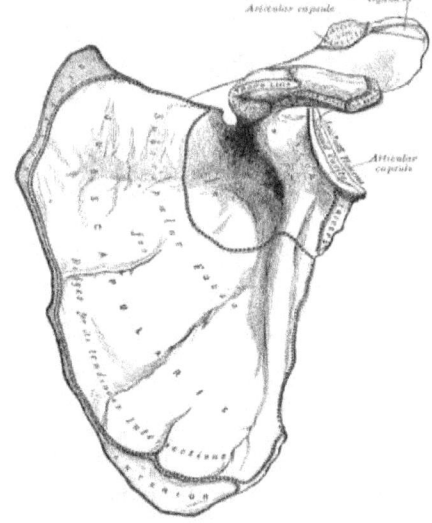

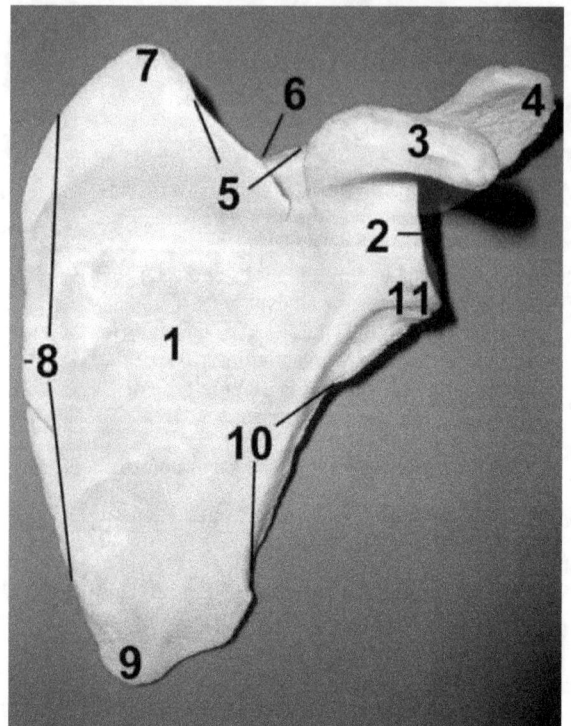

Scapula: Anterior (ventral) surface (Wikipedia.org; Free Encyclopedia).
1 Subscapular fossa. 2 Lateral angle with glenoid cavity. 3 Coracoid process. 4 Acromion process. 5 Superior margin. 6 Suprascapular notch. 7 Superior angle. 8 Medial (vertebral) border. 9 Inferior angle. 10 Lateral border (axillary border). 11 Infraglenoid tubercle.

Table: Vertebral and Rib Levels of the Scapula

Name of the structure	Vertebral level	Rib level	Notes
Spine of the scapula	Third thoracic vertebral spine		The spine of the scapula meets the medial border of the scapula medially and continues as the acromion process laterally
Inferior angle of the scapula	Seventh thoracic vertebral spine	Lower border of the seventh rib Upper part of the seventh intercostals space	The inferior angle is the point where the vertebral border and lateral border meet. The inferior angle of the scapula is subcutaneous and easily palpable.
Scapula		Second to seventh rib	

Note: 1. The lateral and posterior border of the acromion unite to form the **acromion angle**. The medial border of the acromion articulates with the lateral end of the clavicle to form the **acromioclavicular joint**.

2. The **pectoral girdle** is formed by the clavicle and scapula.
3. The **medial border** (vertebral border) of the scapula is thin and it runs parallel to and approximately 5 cm. lateral to the spinous processes of the thoracic vertebrae.
4. The lateral border (**axillary border**) is thick and it runs superolaterally from the inferior angle of the scapula to the axilla at the truncated **lateral angle** of the scapula. The lateral border of the scapula bears **the head of the scapula** at its upper part. The head of the scapula forms the shallow **glenoid cavity**.

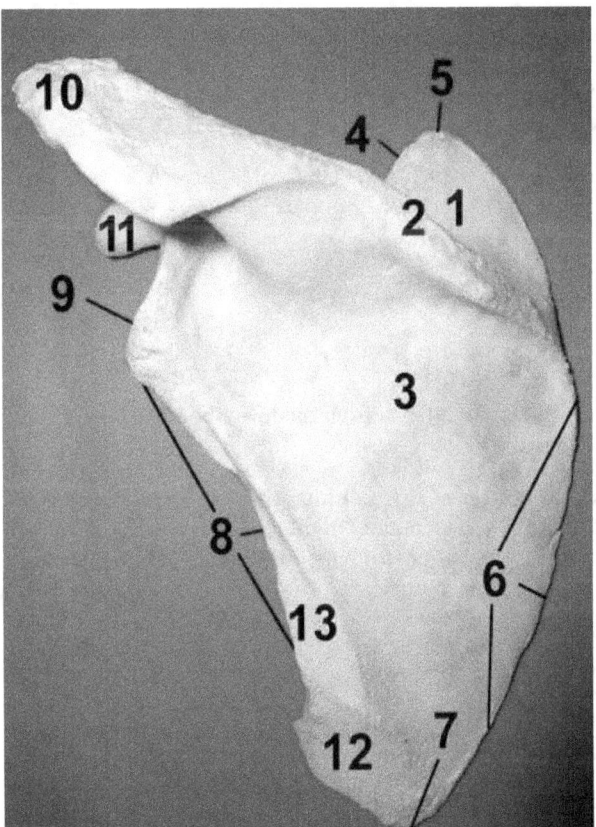

Left scapula: Posterior (dorsal) surface.

(Wikipedia.org; Free Encyclopedia)

1 Supraspinous fossa. 2 Spine of scapula. 3 Infraspinous fossa. 4 Superior border. 5 Superior angle. 6 Medial (vertebral) border. 7 Inferior angle. 8 Lateral border. 9 Lateral angle. 10 Acromion process. 11 Coracoid process. 12 Origin of teres major muscle. and 13 Origin of teres minor muscle.

Lateral Angle of the Scapula (head)

It bears the glenoid cavity. The glenoid cavity forms the glenohumeral joint with the head of the humerus. **The glenohumeral joint is a ball and socket type of synovial joint.**

The supraglenoid tubercle is a small rough area over the glenoid cavity. The supraglenoid tubercle is the site of origin of long head of the biceps brachii muscle**.**

The infraglenoid tubercle is also a small rough area just below the glenoid cavity. The infraglenoid tubercle is the site of origin of the long head of triceps brachii muscle.

The **glenoid fossa (also called glenoid cavity)** is covered by hyaline articular cartilage. The outer part of the glenoid fossa has glenoidal labrum (fibrocartilage) which deepens the socket of the glenohumeral joint to accommodate the large ball (the head of the humerus). **The glenohumeral joint is a ball and socket type of synovial joint.**

The glenohumeral ligaments are three fibrous bands attached to the anterior margin of the glenoid cavity and reinforce the anterior part of the joint capsule.

Lateral Border of the Scapula

The lateral border of the scapula is thick and extends from the lower border of the glenoid cavity to the inferior angle of the scapula.

Origins of muscles from the lateral border of the scapula—1. Long head of biceps brachii (from the infraglenoid tubercle) 2. Teres minor (from the upper two third of the dorsal aspect of the lateral border) 3. Teres major (from the lower third of the dorsal aspect of the lateral border) and 4. Subscapularis (from the costal surface of the lateral border and medial two-thirds of subscapular fossa)

- Thus the lateral border separates the origins of the subscapularis and teres major and minor.

Supraglenoid tubercle of the scapula is located above the glenoid cavity and gives origin to the long head of biceps brachii muscle.

Inferior angle of the scapula is usually at the level of the 7th thoracic spine. It is palpable.

Superior angle of the scapula is **not palpable** because it is covered by the trapezius muscle.

Joints formed by the scapula---1. Glenohumeral joint (shoulder joint) 2. Acromioclavicular joint and 3. Coracoclavicular joint

The Physiological Scapulothoracic Joint

This is the joint between the thoracic wall and the scapula. It provides the basis from which the upper limb functions, allowing the arm to move freely. The scapulothoracic joint has the following movements 1. Elevation-Depression 2. Protraction-Retraction 3. Upward rotation and 4. Downward rotation

Movements of the scapula

Movement of the scapula	Muscles producing movements	Notes
Elevation	**Trapezius(upper part)**, Levator scapulae, and Rhomboids	
Depression	Pectoralis major, Pectoralis minor, Serratus anterior, Trapezius(lower part), Latissimus dorsi, and **Gravity**	
Protraction	**Serratus anterior**, Pectoralis major, and Pectoralis minor	
Retraction	**Trapezius(intermediate part)**, Rhomboids, and Latissimus dorsi	
Upward rotation	**Trapeziums and Serratus anterior**	The glenoid cavity moves superiorly as in abduction of the arm
Downward rotation	**Latissimus dorsi,** Pectoralis major, Pectoralis minor, and Gravity	The glenoid cavity moves inferiorly, as in adduction of the arm

Ligaments Attached to the Scapula

The main scapular ligaments are the 1. **Coracoacromial** and 2. **Superior transverse scapular ligament**.

There may be a weaker, variable inferior transverse scapular ligament (also called **spinoglenoid ligament**). Spinoglenoid ligament is a membranous ligament which may extend from the lateral border of the spine of the scapula to the glenoid margin. It forms an arch over the suprascapular nerve and vessels entering the infraspinous fossa.

Objective Questions

Q.1. Name the articulations of the scapula.

Q.2. Name the ligaments attached to the scapula.

Q.3. Name the origin, insertion, nerve supply, actions of the muscles attached to the scapula.

Q.4. Name the bursae associated with scapula. Which bursa communicates with the shoulder joint?

MCQ

Which of the following muscles takes origin from the subscapular fossa and costal surface of the lateral border of the scapula, adducts and medially rotates the arm, helps hold humeral head in glenoid cavity and is innervated by the upper and lower subscapular nerves?

A. Teres minor

B. Teres major

C. Subscapularis

D. Serratus anterior

The Clavicle

The clavicle is an atypical **long bone**, placed transversely across the neck from the manubrium sterni to the acromion process of the scapula. The bone is subcutaneous and curved, the medial $2/3^{rd}$ is convex anteriorly, and the lateral $1/3^{rd}$ is concave anteriorly. It has two ends, acromial (lateral) and sternal (medial).The anterosuperior surface of the clavicle is **palpable** throughout its length.

The clavicle is also called **collar bone** or beauty bone.

Anatomical position and side determination

1. The flat acromial end of the clavicle lies laterally and articulates with the medial side of the acromion process of scapula.

2. The rounded sternal end lies medially and articulates with the manubrium sterni.

3. The shaft is convex in its medial two-thirds and concave forward in its lateral one third.

4. The undersurface of the middle third of the clavicular shaft presents the subclavian groove.

Sex differences of clavicle

Female clavicle	Male clavicle
Shorter, thinner, less curved and smoother and its acromial end is carried lower than the sternal end.	The acromial end is on level, with or slightly higher than, the sternal end when the arm is in anatomical position.

Note: The clavicle is thicker and more curved in manual workers, and its ridges for muscular attachment are more distinct.

Functions of the Clavicle

1. It acts as a cross-piece for keeping the upper limb away from the trunk and permits the limb the optimum range of motion.

2. It transmits forces from the upper extremity to the trunk.

3. It is an essential component of the shoulder girdle.

4. The clavicle connects the pectoral girdle and the axial skeleton.

5. The clavicle is the only bony attachment between the upper limb and trunk.

Peculiarities of the Clavicle

1. The clavicle has no medullary cavity.

2. It is mostly intramembranous in ossification.

3. It is the first bone to begin ossification in the body, but it is last to complete ossification*.

4. It is the only long bone with two primary centers of ossification.

5. It is infrequently pierced by the middle supraclavicular nerve.

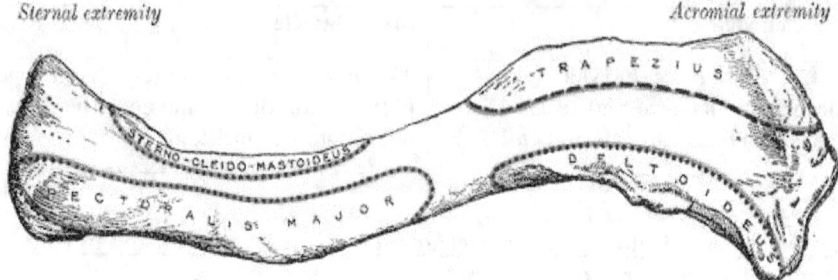

Figure: Muscle attachments to superior surface of left clavicle

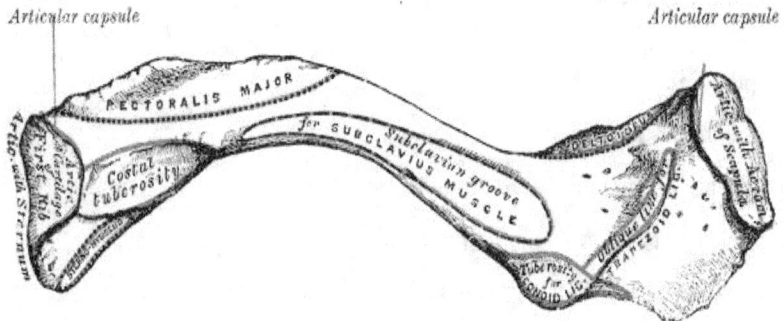

Figure: Muscle attachments to the inferior surface of left clavicle

(Wikipedia.org; Free Encyclopedia)

Ossification of the Clavicle

The clavicle is the bone, which begins to **ossify first** in the body. The entire clavicle develops from **intramembranous ossification** with the exception of the medial end that develops from intracartilaginous ossification. It has **two primary centers** and one **secondary center** of ossification. The primary centers emerge in the shaft during 5th to 6th weeks of intrauterine life and unites about the 45th day. A secondary center emerges at the medial end during 15-17 years and fuses with the shaft during **21-22 years.** The clavicle completes ossification last in the body.

Note: The ossification of the clavicle begins in the 5th week of intrauterine life but it is completed at about the 21st year.

Attachments of Clavicle

Muscles and ligaments that attach to the clavicle include:

Attachment on clavicle	Muscle/Ligament	Site of attachment
Superior surface and anterior border	Deltoid muscle(origin)	deltoid tubercle, anteriorly on the lateral third of clavicle
Superior surface	Trapezius muscle	posteriorly on the lateral third of clavicle
Inferior surface	Subclavius muscle(insertion)	subclavian groove of the clavicle
Inferior surface	Conoid ligament (the medial part of the coracoclavicular ligament)	conoid tubercle of the clavicle
Inferior surface	Trapezoid ligament (the lateral part of the coracoclavicular ligament)	trapezoid line of the clavicle
Anterior border	Pectoralis major muscle	medial third (rounded border) of clavicle
Posterior border	Sternocleidomastoid muscle (clavicular head)	superiorly, on the medial third of clavicle
Posterior border	Sternohyoid muscle	inferiorly, on the medial third of the clavicle
Posterior border	Trapezius muscle	lateral third of the clavicle

Medial end of the clavicle gives attachment to the 1. Sternoclavicular 2. Interclavicular and costoclavicular ligaments.

Lateral end of the clavicle gives attachment to the acromioclavicular ligament.

*The **subclavian groove** is located on the inferior surface of the middle third of the clavicle. It gives insertion to the subclavius muscle and attachment to the clavipectoral fascia.

A **nutrient foramen** is found in the lateral part of the subclavian groove, running in a lateral direction. Hence, the medial end of the clavicle is the growing end. The nutrient artery of the clavicle is derived from the suprascapular artery.

Structures located along the posterior surface of the medial 2/3rd of the clavicle (from medial to lateral)

1. Lower end of the internal jugular vein separated by the sternohyoid muscle.

2. Junction of the subclavian vein with the internal jugular vein forming the brachiocephalic vein.

3. Trunks of brachial plexus

4. Third part of subclavian artery

5. Suprascapular vessels

Congenital Anomaly: Ceidocranial dysostosis

A congenital anomaly characterized by absence of clavicle, enlarged incompletely ossified skull with frontal protuberance, and poor teeth formation.

Congenital Anomaly: Poland syndrome

A congenital anomaly characterized by absence of pectoralis major and minor, deficient development of 2-4 ribs, and breast hypoplasia,

Objective Question

Q. How is the clavicle different from other long bones? What structures could be damaged with a clavicular fracture?

Notes: The clavicle is usually **fractured** medial to the conoid tubercle because the middle third of the bone is not strengthened with ligaments and muscles. (Wikipedia.org; Free Encyclopedia)

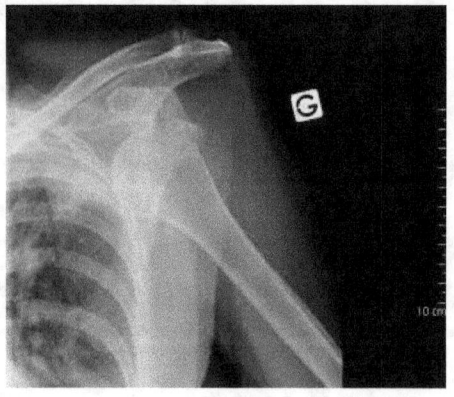 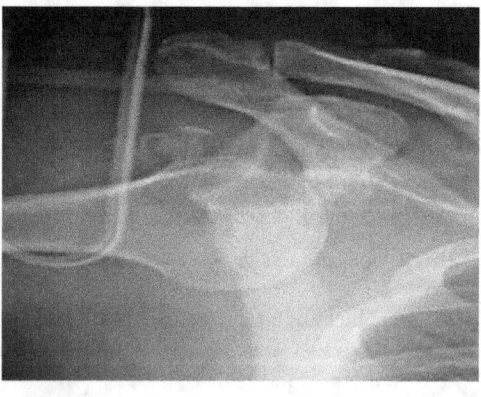

Figure: Anterior dislocation of shoulder   Figure: Inferior dislocation of shoulder

Joints of the Pectoral Region

Name of the joint & articulating bones	Type of joint	Movements and muscles acting on the joint	Nerve supply	Blood supply	Accessory structures
Sternoclavicular joint **Articulating surfaces** Medial end(sternal end) of the clavicle and the clavicular notch of the manubrium sterni and the costal cartilage of the first rib	Saddle type of synovial joint(articular surfaces are concavoconvex)	Elevation and depression, abduction and adduction, protraction and retraction, flexion and , and circumduction	Medial supraclavicular nerve Nerve to the subclavius	Internal thoracic artery Suprascapular artery	Fibrous capsule Costoclavicular ligament Articular disc Interclavicular ligament Anterior and posterior sternoclavicular ligaments
Acromioclavicular joint **Articulating surfaces** Acromial end (lateral end) of the clavicle and the medial acromial margin	Plane type of synovial joint	Elevation and depression, abduction and adduction, protraction and retraction, flexion and circumduction	Suprascapular nerve Lateral pectoral nerve	Surascapular artery Thoracoacromial arteries	Acromioclavicular ligament Coracoclavicular ligament

Shoulder joint (glenohumeral joint) Articulating surfaces	Ball and socket type of synovial joint	**Flexion:** **Pectoralis major** and anterior fiber of deltoid, corocobrachialis, short head of biceps brachii **Extension** **Posterior fibers of deltoid**, and teres major, **Adduction:** **Pectoralis major, latissimus dorsi,** subscapularis, infraspinatus, and teres minor **Abduction:** **Deltoid,** and supraspinatus **Medial rotation:** **Subscapularis,** Pectoralis major, anterior fibers of deltoid, and latissimus dorsi **Lateral rotation:** **Infraspinatus,**teres minor, and posterior fibers of deltoid	Axillary nerve Suprascapular nerve Musculocutaneous nerve	Anterior circumflex humeral artery Posterior circumflex humeral artery Suprascapular artery Subscapular artery	Fibrous capsule Coracohumeral ligament Transverse humeral ligament Glenoidal labrum

Notes:

Testing abduction, medial, and lateral rotation of the humerus at the **shoulder joint tests motor function mainly of spinal levels C5 and C6.**

The pectoral (shoulder) girdle is a bony ring, deficient posteriorly, formed by the scapulae and clavicles and completed anteriorly by the manubrium of the sternum.

The articular cavity of the **sternoclavicular joint** is completely separated into two compartments by a fibrocartilaginous articular disc. Superiorly, the disc is firmly attached to the upper part of the medial end of the clavicle. Inferiorly, the disc is firmly attached to the upper part of the first costal cartilage. The articular disc prevents medial displacement of the clavicle. The articular disc and the associated ligaments maintain the stability of the sternoclavicular joint.

Dislocation of the sternoclavicular joint is rare although **fracture of clavicle** is common. Fracture of the clavicle usually occurs near the junction of its middle and lateral thirds.

Fracture of the clavicle

The clavicle is the single bone attachment between the upper limb and trunk. Because it is involved with conveying forces from the upper limb to the trunk, it can easily be fractured.

The clavicle is one of the most commonly fractured bones. Usually the junction between the lateral and middle third of the clavicle is the site of fracture because the middle third of the clavicle is not reinforced with ligaments or muscles. The proximal fragment of the clavicle is displaced upwards because of the pull of the **sternocleidomastoid** muscle. The distal fragment moves downwards and medially because of gravity **and the pull of the pectoralis major muscle. Overriding of the clavicle pieces shorten the clavicle. A clavicular fracture** can produce neurovascular damage because major **neurovascular structures** like the subclavian vessels and lower trunk of the **brachial plexus** lie between the clavicle and the first rib (Wikipedia.org; Free Encyclopedia).

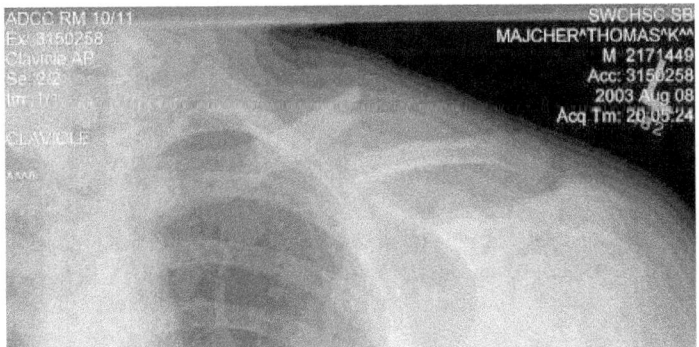

Movement at the sternoclavicular joint is vital to the movement of the shoulder joint. Hence ankylosis of the sternoclavicular joint needs surgical intervention in order to maintain movements of the shoulder joint.

Movements at the acromioclavicular and the sternoclavicular joints are passive. No muscles directly move the joints, but muscles which move the scapula indirectly move the clavicle. There is a close interaction between the scapulae and clavicles; hence, a fractured clavicle affects the movement of the scapula.

The articulating surfaces of the **acromioclavicular joint** are covered by **fibrocartilage**. An **articular disc** is often present in the acromioclavicular joint.

The Coracoclavicular Ligament

The coracoclavicular ligament connects the **superior surface of the coracoid process** of the scapula and the lower surface of the **lateral part of the clavicle.** Although not in direct contact with the acromioclavicular joint, **it is very important to maintain the stability of the acromioclavicular joint.** The coracoclavicular ligament has conoid and trapezoid parts, often separated by fat and a bursa.

The **conoid ligament** is conical with its apex attaches to the root of the coracoid process near the suprascapular notch and its base attaches to the inferior surface of the lateral part of the clavicle.

The **trapezoid ligament** is **lateral** to the conoid ligament. It attaches to the superior surface of the coracoid process and extends laterally and superiorly to the trapezoid line on the inferior surface of the lateral part of the clavicle. The weight of the upper limb is passed on from the scapula to the clavicle through the coracoclavicular ligament, and from the clavicle to the sternum through the sternoclavicular joint.

The coracoclavicular ligament is a **much stronger** attachment between the clavicle and scapula than the acromioclavicular joint is. In a clavicular fracture medial to the coracoclavicular ligament, the **"shoulder"** goes down.

Dislocation of the Acromioclavicular Joint

This is common because the acromioclavicular joint is weak. A dislocation may happen during body contact sports or a fall on the shoulder or outstretched hand. An acromioclavicular dislocation is commonly called a "**shoulder separation**". Shoulder separation is associated with acromioclavicular and coracoclavicular ligament damage. In coracoclavicular ligament damage, the shoulder separates from the clavicle and goes down because of the weight of the upper limb (shoulder droop). The fibrous capsule of the acromioclavicular joint may be damaged so that the acromion can pass underneath the lateral end of the clavicle.

Bursae related to the glenohumeral joint

1. Subacromial or subdeltoid bursa, does not communicate with the glenohumeral joint cavity

2. Subscapularis bursa, communicates with the glenohumeral joint cavity.

3. Infraspinatus bursa, may communicate with the glenohumeral joint cavity

Clinical note:

Frozen Shoulder (adhesive capsulitis of the glenohumeral joint)

Frozen shoulder occurs when the connective tissue (e.g., joint capsule, rotator cuff or subacromial bursa) enclosing the shoulder joint becomes thickened and tight. Usually the patient is of 40-60 years of age, with history of prolonged immobilization of the upper limb as seen in fracture, or dislocation of bones. It may be seen in diabetic or ischemic heart disease patients and sometimes the cause is unknown. A patient with this condition has difficulty abducting the arm. Frozen shoulder can be managed by stretch exercises to improve the range of motion of the shoulder joint.

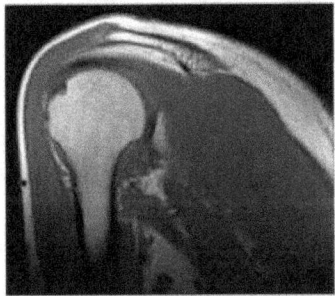

Fig. MRI of Frozen Shoulder (Right) showing thickening of supraspinatus tendon

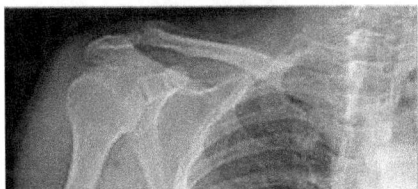

Fig. Plane X-Ray of right shoulder joint of the same patient (without any abnormalities)

Objective Questions

1. What is the most common site of clavicle fracture? Why?

2. Why does the distal portion of the clavicle drop below the proximal fragment?

MCQ

1. Which of the following bones is the only bony attachment between the upper limb and the trunk?

A. Scapula

B. Humerus

C. Sternum

D. Clavicle

The Humerus

The humerus is a cylindrical **long bone** which forms the skeleton of the arm or brachium.

The Head of the Humerus

The head of the humerus is smooth and hemispherical in form. It is separated from the shaft by the **anatomical neck**. It has two palpable **tuberosities** separated by an **intertubercular groove**. It is covered by hyaline articular cartilage in life. It articulates with the glenoid fossa of the scapula to form the shoulder joint.

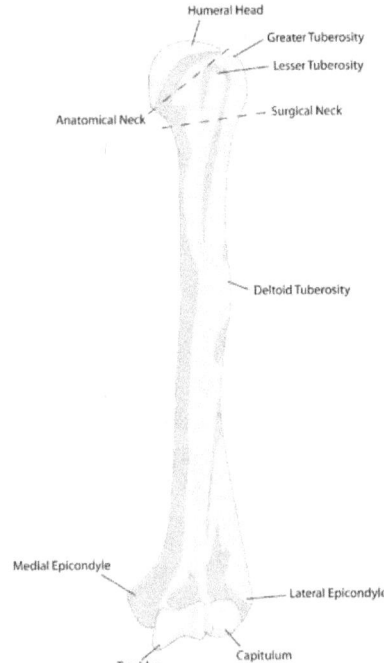

Figure: The anterior view of the humerus

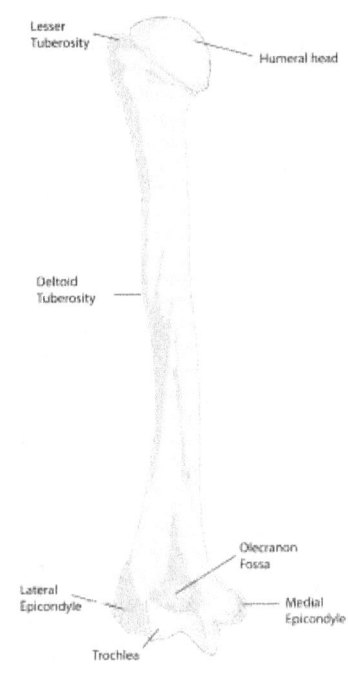

Figure: The posterior view of the humerus

(Wikipedia.org; Free Encyclopedia)

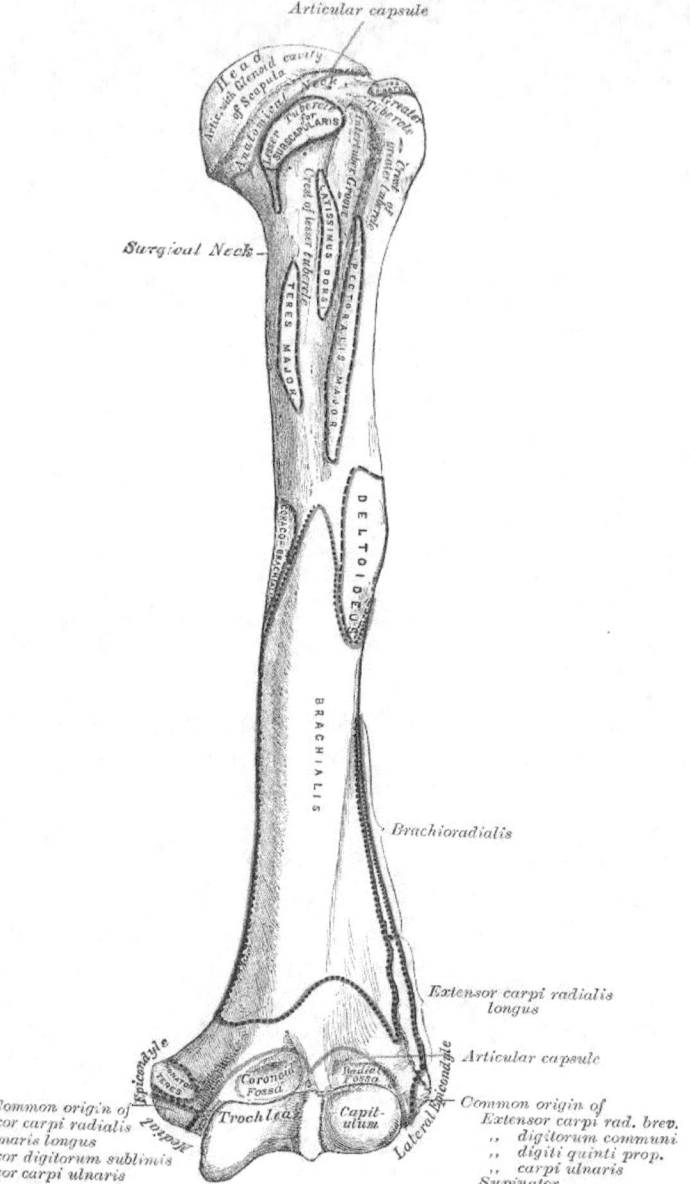

Figure: Anterior view of the humerus

(Wikipedia.org; Free Encyclopedia)

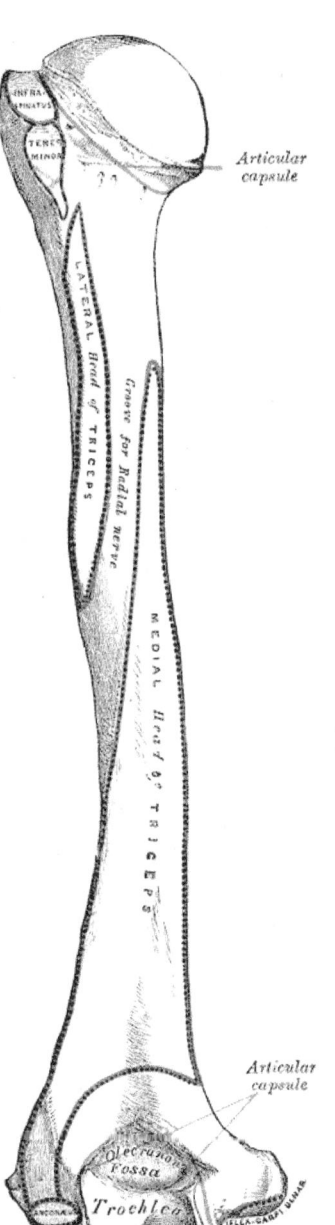

Figure:

Posterior view of the humerus
(Wikipedia.org; Free Encyclopedia)

The Epiphyseal Lines of Humerus

The epiphyseal line of the humerus is the site of fusion of epiphysis with metaphysis. It remains cartilaginous until the bone reaches its adult size between 19th and 21st years. When growth stops, the epiphyseal plate is replaced by a synostosis (bone to bone fusion), seen as an epiphyseal line in X-Rays.

Each humerus has a proximal and a distal epiphyseal line.

The diaphysis develops from a primary center of ossification. A primary center of ossification appears during intrauterine life (8th week of development).

The Greater Tubercle of the Humerus

It is located on the outer aspect of the upper end of the humerus.

It bears three impressions for tendinous insertion of three muscles on its posterosuperior aspect.

Its medial margin forms the lateral part of the bicipital groove (intertubercular sulcus).

Attachments of the Greater Tubercle of the Humerus—insertion of three muscles

1. Supraspinatus—on the uppermost impression; 2. Infraspinatus on middle impression and; 3. Teres minor on lowest impression

The transverse humeral ligament bridges the greater and lesser tubercle of the humerus for the passage of the tendon of the long head of the biceps brachii.

The greater tubercle is covered by the deltoid muscle. The subacromial bursa may extend between the deltoid muscle and the greater tubercle of the humerus.

The Lesser Tubercle of the Humerus

It is situated in front of the head just below the anatomical neck and forms the medial border of the intertubercular sulcus (bicipital groove).

Attachments

1. Insertion of subscapularis muscle; 2. Attachment of transverse humeral ligament

The Intertubercular Sulcus (bicipital groove or intertubercular groove)

This is a groove between the greater and lesser tubercle of the humerus on the anterior surface of the upper part of the humerus. It has a medial lip, a lateral lip and the floor between the lips.

Muscular insertions to the bicipital groove—1.Pectoralis major to the lateral lip 2.Teres major to the medial lip and; 3. Latissimus dorsi to the floor

Contents of the Bicipital Groove

1. Tendon of long head of biceps brachii and its synovial sheath

2. An ascending branch from the anterior circumflex humeral artery

Muscular Attachments to the Anterior Surface of the Shaft of the Humerus

Insertions of—1. Deltoid muscle to the anterolateral surface of the middle of the shaft of the humerus (**deltoid tuberosity**), 2. Coracobrachialis muscle to the anteromedial surface of the middle of the shaft of the humerus.

Origins of ---1. Brachialis from the lower half of the anterior, anteromedial, and anterolateral surface of the humerus, 2. Origin of brachioradialis from the lateral supracondylar line.

Surgical Neck of the Humerus

The proximal end of the humerus joins the shaft at an ill-defined 'surgical neck', **just below the greater and lesser tubercles**.

Relations of the medial side of the surgical neck of the humerus

1. Axillary nerve and 2. Posterior circumflex humeral artery

* The surgical neck of the humerus is a common site of fracture.

Anatomical Neck of the Humerus

The anatomical neck of the humerus is a slight constriction adjoining the margin of the head. The anatomical neck of the humerus is the line of capsular attachment of the shoulder joint other than at the intertubercular sulcus, where the long tendon of biceps brachii emerges. Medially, the capsular attachment moves away from the anatomical neck and descends 1cm or more onto the shaft.

Shaft of the Humerus

The shaft or diaphysis of the humerus is tubular in its upper half while it is triangular and flattened below. It has three borders---1. Anterior, 2. Lateral and,3. Medial . The shaft of the humerus has three surfaces—1. Anterolateral; 2. Anteromedial and; 3. Posterior

Attachment to the **medial border** of the middle of the shaft of the humerus is the insertion of the **coracobrachialis** muscle.

The **deltoid tuberosity** is a V-shaped rough area at the middle of the anterolateral surface of the shaft of the humerus for the insertion of the deltoid muscle.

The **brachialis** muscle takes origin from the lower half of the anterior, anterolateral, and anteromedial surface of the shaft of the humerus.

The oblique **radial or spiral groove** is situated on the middle of the **posterior surface** of the humerus between the origin of the lateral and medial heads of the triceps brachii muscle. The radial or spiral groove contains the radial nerve and profunda brachii artery.

The posterior surface also contains the **nutrient foramen** for the nutrient artery, which is derived from brachial or profunda brachii artery. The nutrient foramen is directed towards the elbow because the upper end is the growing end of the humerus.

Objective Question

Q. 1. What artery accompanies the radial nerve in the spiral groove?

Q.2. Nutrient artery of the humerus is a branch of which artery?

Muscular Attachments of the Posterior Surface of the Humerus

1. Lateral head of triceps brachii---arises from the oblique line above the radial groove

2. Medial head of triceps brachii---arises from the posterior surface of the shaft of the humerus below the radial groove.

Capitulum

The capitulum is the lateral, convex, and rounded lower articular part of the humerus. It articulates with the head of the radius forming the humero-radial component of the elbow joint.

Trochlea

The trochlea is a **pulley-shaped** medial part of the lower end of the humerus. It is separated from the capitulum by a groove. The trochlea articulates with the trochlear notch of the ulna forming the humero-ulnar component of the elbow joint.

The two margins of the trochlea are of unequal size. The medial margin is deeper and helps in forming the carrying angle.

Carrying angle

It is the angle between the long axis of the humerus and the supinated forearm and hand. The carrying angle is approximately 165° in female and 175° in male.

The distal end of the humerus is a modified condyle.

Nonarticular parts of the lower end of the humerus include medial and lateral epicondyles, olecranon and coronoid and radial fossae. The medial epicondyle is more distinct than the lateral epicondyle.

Medial supracondylar ridge is the lower continuation of the medial border of the humerus. Medial supracondylar ridge ends in the medial epicondyle.

Muscular attachments of the medial epicondyle and medial supracondylar ridge

Common origin of the superficial flexor muscles of the forearm—1. Pronator teres, 2. Flexor carpi radialis, 3. Palmaris longus, 4. Flexor carpi ulnaris, and 5. Flexor digitorum superficialis

The humeral head of the pronator teres originates from the lower part of the medial supracondylar ridge.

Other attachments—1. Ulnar collateral ligament of elbow joint, and 2. Medial intermuscular septum

Muscular attachments to the lateral epicondyle of the humerus:

Common extensor origin for—1. Extensor carpi radialis longus, 2. Extensor carpi radialis brevis, 3. Extensor digitorum, 4.Extensor digiti minimi, and 5. extensor carpi ulnaris

Muscular attachments of lateral supracondylar ridge:

Origins of 1. Brachioradialis, 2. Extensor carpi radialis longus.

The lateral supracondylar ridge also gives attachment to the lateral intermuscular septum. The lateral intermuscular septum is pierced by the radial nerve.

The radial collateral ligament of the elbow is attached to the lateral epicondyle of the humerus.

Fossae

1. Olecranon fossa—is a depression on the posterior aspect of the humerus, just above the trochlea. This fossa houses the olecranon process of the ulna.

2. Coronoid fossa—is a small depression on the anterior aspect of the humerus just above the trochlea. Upon flexion of the forearm, this fossa lodges the coronoid process of the ulna.

3. Radial fossa---is a small depression over the capitulum on the lateral side of the coronoid fossa.Upon flexion of the forearm, it accommodates the head of the radius.

Nerves intimately related to the humerus and their lesions in bony fracture

A. Axillary nerve

Axillary nerve may be involved with fracture of the surgical neck of the humerus.

B. Radial nerve

Radial nerve in the **radial groove (in the middle of the posterior surface of the humerus)** may be involved with **fracture of the shaft of the humerus.**

C. Ulnar nerve

Ulnar nerve may be involved with fractures of the **medial epicondyle** of the humerus.

D. Median nerve

Median nerve may be involved in supracondylar fracture of the humerus.

The Four Most Common Sites of Humeral Fracture:

1. The surgical neck of the humerus

2. The midshaft of the humerus

3. The supracondylar region of the humerus

4. The medial epicondyle of the humerus

Structures related to the posterior aspect of the medial epicondyle of the humerus

1. Ulnar nerve, 2. Superior ulnar collateral artery

Structure related to the anterior aspect of the medial epicondyle of the humerus

1. Inferior ulnar collateral artery

Objective Questions

Q1. Which structures pass to the anterior and posterior aspect of the medial epicondyle?

2. Which nerve may be injured due to fracture of the middle shaft (diaphysis) of the humerus?

MCQs

1. Which of the following nerves would be damaged with injuries to the medial epicondyle of the humerus?

A. Radial nerve

B. Median nerve

C. Ulnar nerve

D. Musculocutaneous nerve

2. Which of the following muscles would be most likely to be paralyzed due to a tear of ulnar nerve near the medial epicondyle of the humerus?

A. Supinator

B. Biceps brachii

C. Brachialis

D. Anconeus

E. Flexor carpi ulnaris

3. Which pair of structures is most likely to be injured due to a fracture at the mid shaft (diasphysis) of the humerus?

A. Radial nerve and profunda brachii artery

B. Median nerve and brachial artery

C. Axillary nerve and posterior humeral circumflex artery

D. Long thoracic nerve and lateral thoracic artery

4. Which nerve is injured by the jagged edges of a broken bone due to transverse fracture of the humerus about 3 cm proximal to the epicondyles?

A. Axillary nerve

B. Median nerve

C. Radial nerve

D. Ulnar nerve

E. Musculocutaneous nerve

Radius and Ulna

These two long bones form the skeleton of the forearm.

Ulna

The ulna is a long bone. It is the medial bone of the forearm. The upper end of the ulna presents the **olecranon and coronoid processes, and the trochlear and radial notches**. The posterior border of the shaft of the ulna is subcutaneous. Therefore, it is likely to be fractured by direct violence (a 'defense' fracture).

Side determination

1. The olecranon process is above.

2. The trochlear notch is in front.

3. The sharp interosseous border lies laterally.

4. The styloid process lies inferomedially.

Olecranon Process of the Ulna—is the uppermost part of the ulna. The olecranon process of the ulna forms the point of the elbow.

Attachment to olecranon

From the medial surface—1. Origin of flexor digitorum profundus, 2. Origin of flexor carpi ulnaris, and 3. Lower end of the ulnar collateral ligament

On the superoposterior surface---1. Insertion of triceps brachii muscle, and 2. Insertion of anconeus muscle,3. Capsule of the elbow joint.

The olecranon process is separated from the subcutaneous tissue by the olecranon bursa. The olecranon bursa may be inflamed (bursitis) due to repeated and prolonged pressure (**students' elbow**).

Olecranon spur—results from ossification in the tendinous insertion of the triceps brachii muscle. It may be visible in an adult plain x-ray of elbow region.

Coronoid Process of the Ulna

The coronoid process projects forward from the shaft of the ulna just below the olecranon process.

Attachment to Coronoid Process of Ulna

Insertion of brachialis muscle

Origins of 1. Flexor digitorum profundus, 2. Pronator teres, 3. Flexor pollicis longus

Attachment of ulnar collateral ligament

Borders of the Ulna

The shaft of the ulna has three borders—1. Anterior, 2. Posterior, and 3. Interosseous

The anterior **border** is thick and rounded. It extends from the ulnar tuberosity to the styloid process of the ulna.

The **interosseous border** is sharp. The radioulnar interosseous membrane is attached to the interosseous border of the ulna

Posterior Border of the Ulna

The posterior border of the ulna is **subcutaneous**. It extends from the olecranon process to the styloid process of the ulna. The posterior border of the ulna provides the aponeurotic origins of the 1. Flexor carpi ulnaris, 2. Extensor carpi ulnaris, and 3. Flexor digitorum profundus.

Radial Notch of Ulna

Radial notch of the ulna is a small, oval depression on the upper part of the lateral surface of the coronoid process. The radial notch articulates with the head of the radius to form the superior radioulnar joint. Superior radioulnar joint is a pivot type of synovial joint.

Radius

The radius is the lateral bone of the forearm.

Side determination

1. The disc like head of the radius is above.

2. The gentle concavity of the shaft is in front.

3. The styloid process lies inferolaterally.

Radial Tuberosity

The radial tuberosity is situated just below the medial part of the neck of the radius. It has a rough posterior part for the insertion of biceps brachii and smooth anterior part covered by a bursa.

Neck of the Radius

It is the constriction immediately below the head. This is the cylindrical region between the expanded head and the radial tuberosity. The neck is enclosed by the narrow, lower margin of the annular ligament.

Head of the Radius

The head is circular and is covered by hyaline articular cartilage. Its superior surface is concave and articulates with the capitulum of the humerus at the elbow joint. The circumference of the head articulates with the radial notch of the ulna to form the superior radioulnar joint.

The Distal End of the Radius

The distal end of the radius is wide and quadrangular. Its medial aspect has the **ulnar notch** to accommodate the head of the ulna. Its lateral aspect extends distally as the **radial styloid process.** A palpable **dorsal tubercle** of the radius is located on the dorsal aspect. There is a groove on the medial part of the dorsal tubercle for the passage of the tendon of the **extensor pollicis longus.**

The Interosseous Border of the Radius and Ulna

It is the site of attachment of the interosseous membrane. The fibers of the interosseous membrane pass downwards and medially from the radius to ulna. Therefore, **forces received by the radius (via the hand) are transmitted to the ulna and then to the humerus.**

Elbow Joint

The elbow joint is a hinge type of synovial joint. The elbow joint consists of articulations among three bones: the humerus, radius, and ulna.

1. Humeroulnar joint

A. The humeroulnar joint is strengthened by the ulnar (medial) collateral ligament.

B. A tear of ulnar collateral ligament will allow unusual abduction of the forearm.

2. Humeroradial joint

A. The radiohumeral joint is strengthened by the radial collateral ligament.

B. A tear of radial collateral ligament will allow unusual adduction of the forearm.

Note: The elbow joint is continuous with the superior radioulnar joint.

Elbow radiographs

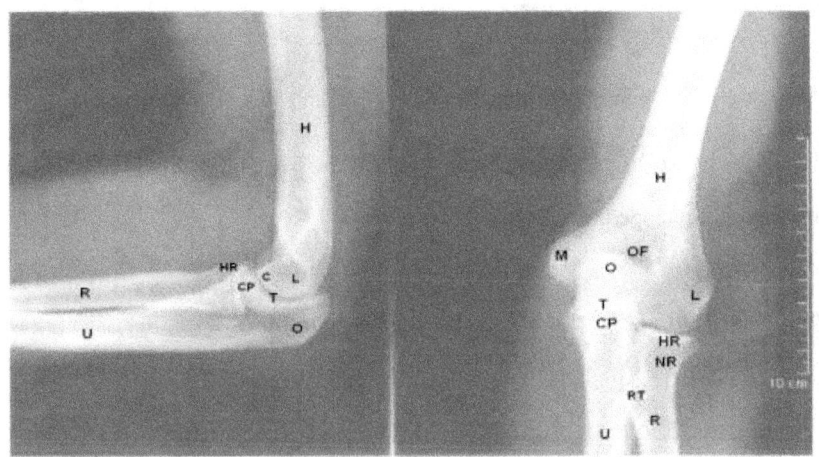

Lateral radiograph   **Anteroposterior radiograph**

(Wikipedia.org; Free Encyclopedia)

C Capitulum, **CP** Coronoid process of ulna, **H** Humerus , **HR** Head of radius, **L** Lateral epicondyle, **O** Olecranon, **R** Radius, **T** Trochlear notch, **U** Ulna, **NR** Neck of radius, **OF** Olecranon fossa, **T** Trochlea of humerus, **RT** Radial tuberosity, **U** Ulna.

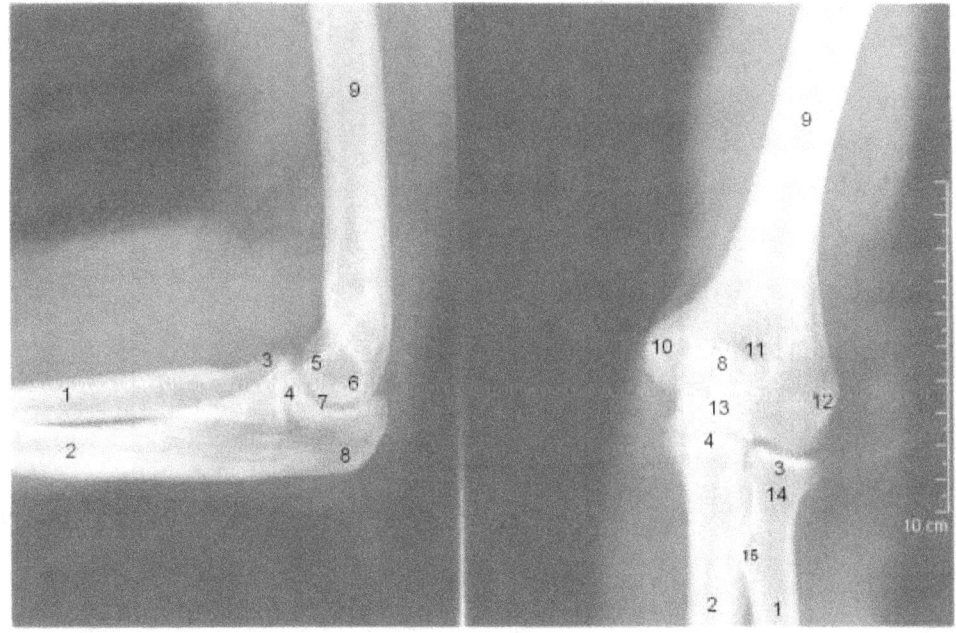

Lateral radiograph   **Anteroposterior radiograph**

1) Radius, 2) Ulna, 3) Head of radius, 4) Coronoid process, 5) Capitulum, 6) Lateral epicondyle
7) Trochlear notch, 8) Olecranon process, 9) Humerus, 10) Medial epicondyle, 11) Olecranon
fossa, 12) Medial epicondyle, 13) Trochlea, 14) Neck of radius, 15) Radial tuberosity

(Wikipedia.org; Free Encyclopedia)

Elbow Joint/Superior Radioulnar Joint/Inferior Radioulnar Joint

Name of the joint and articulating bones	Type of joint	Movements and muscles acting on the joint	Nerve supply	Blood supply	Ligaments
Elbow joint **Articulating surfaces** The capitulum and trochlea of the humerus, upper surface of the head of the radius, and trochlear notch of the ulna	Hinge type of synovial joint	1. **Flexion** is brought about by the –1. Brachialis, 2. Biceps Brachii, and 3. Brachioradial is **2. Extension** is brought about by the –1.Triceps brachii and 2. Anconeus	1. Ulnar nerve 2. Median nerve 3.Radial nerve 4. Musculocutaneous nerve	From anastomosis around the elbow joint	1. Capsular ligament 2.Ulnar collateral ligament 3. Radial collateral ligament
Superior radioulnar joint **Articulating surfaces** Circumference of head of radius Radial notch	Pivot type of synovial joint	**Supination** is brought about by the 1. Supinator and Biceps brachii **Pronation** is brought about by the 1.Pronator	1.Musculocutaneous 2. Radial and 3. Median and 4. Ulnar nerves	Anastomos is around the elbow joint	1.Annular ligament 2. Quadrate ligament

of ulna		quadratus and 2. Pronator teres			
Inferior radioulnar joint **Articulating surfaces** Convex distal head of the ulna Concave ulnar notch of the radius	Pivot type of synovial joint	**Supination** is brought about by the 1. Supinator and Biceps brachii **Pronation** is brought about by the 1.Pronator quadratus and 2. Pronator teres	1. Anterior interosseous nerve 2. Posterior interosseous nerve	1. Anterior interosseou s artery 2. Posterior interosseou s artery	

Lesions around the Elbow Joint/ Secondary Ossification Centers Around the Elbow

The elbow joint area is a common site of fracture. In an adult it is easy to read the lateral and anterior- posterior radiograph, but in children additional factors require interpretation. In children, multiple secondary ossification centers appear before and around puberty. The approximate ages of **emergence of secondary ossification centers around the elbow joint are**:

Capitulum----1 year

Medial epicondyle----5 years

Head of radius----5 years

Trochlea----11 years

Olecranon process----12 years

Lateral epicondyle----13 years

Supracondylar fracture of the distal part of the humerus is, as a rule, seen in children following a fall on the outstretched hand. The distal fragment is commonly displaced posteriorly. The serrated end of the proximal fragment can sometimes injure the **brachial artery and or the median nerve.**

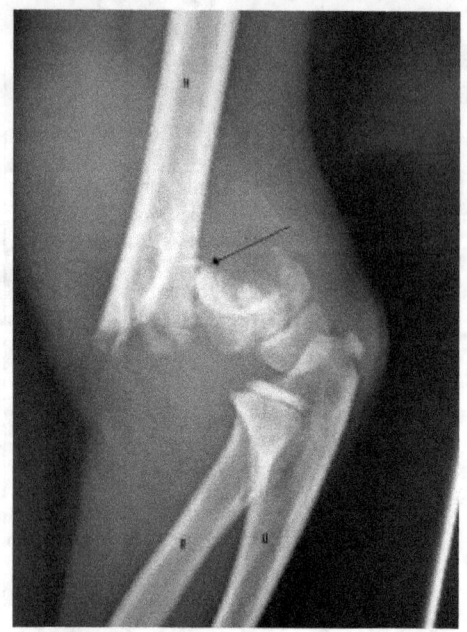

Figure: An elbow x-ray showing a supracondylar fracture in a young child (H = humerus. **R** = Radius. **U** = Ulna. Fracture is marked by an arrow). (Wikipedia.org; Free Encyclopedia)

Elbow Arthritis

Osteoarthritis of the elbow joint is very common. A chronic degenerative process, in which small bony fragments may appear in the relatively small articular cavity, can result in limitation of movements of the elbow joint.

Epicondylitis

Overuse strain of the common flexor origin from the medial epicondyle of the humerus may cause pain on the medial epicondyle. This is typically seen in golf players **(Golfer's elbow).**

Overuse strain of the common extensor origin from the lateral epicondyle of the humerus may cause pain on the lateral epicondyle. This is typically seen in tennis players **(Tennis elbow).**

Traumatic Dislocation of the Elbow Joint

Posterior dislocation of the elbow joint with ulnar abduction is often complicated by fracture of the coronoid process. The brachial artery and /or median and ulnar nerves can occasionally be damaged along with separation of the medial epicondyle.This type of injury is common along with supracondylar fracture of the distal humerus.

Pulled elbow/Nursemaid's Elbow

Subluxation or dislocation of the radial head through the annular ligament due to a sudden pull on the arm is a relatively common injury in young children. The child may cry out, dislikes to use the limb and hold the upper limb with elbow flexed and forearm pronated.This type of injury is common in children because the annular ligament has vertical sides in children compared with more funnel shaped sides in adult. This is uncommon after the age of five because the head of the radius begins to ossify and is no longer deformable.

Reduction includes forcefully supinating and flexing the elbow, which snaps the ligament back into place.

Objective Questions

Q.1. Explain why elbow dislocations are more likely to occur in the children.

Q.2. Which bones articulate to form the elbow joint?

Q. 3. Name the movements at the elbow joint? What specific muscles are involved in each of the movements?

Distal Radius and Ulna

Greenstick fracture of the radius and ulna is the bowing or splintering at the site of incomplete fracture. It is commonly seen in young children.

Colles fracture involves the distal part of the radius with posterior displacement of the distal radius. A typical **dinner fork** deformity is commonly seen in **elderly women**. The distal part of the radius may be broken into pieces with associated ulnar avulsion.

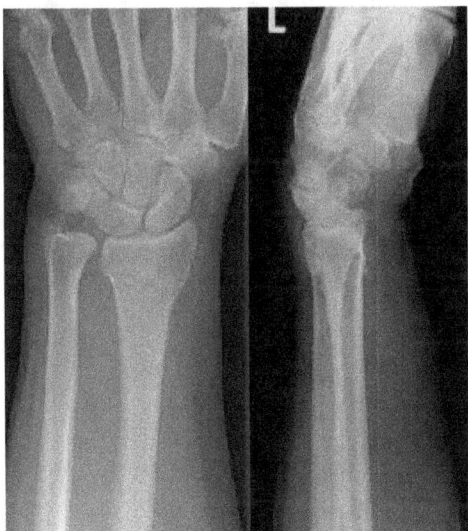

Figure: Colles fracture (Wikipedia.org; Free Encyclopedia).

Carpal Bones

Proximal row: (**S**he **L**ooks **T**oo **P**retty)—1. **S**caphoid 2. **L**unate 3. **T**riquetrum 4. **P**isiform

Distal row: (**Try** **to** **C**atch **H**er) -----------2. **T**rapezium 2. **T**rapezoid 3. **C**apitate 4. **H**amate

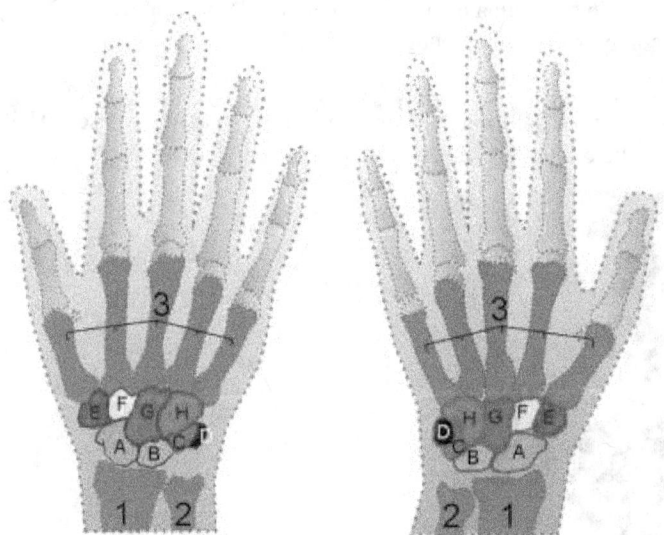

Proximal:

- A-Scaphoid
- B-Lunate
- C-Triquetrum (Triangular)
- D-Pisiform

Distal:

- E-Trapezium
- F-Trapezoid

- G-Capitate
- H-Hamate

  3 –indicates the metacarpals 1 through 5

(Wikipedia.org; Free Encyclopedia)

Scaphoid

The scaphoid is a boat-shaped bone. Its long axis is oblique and has a tubercle on its lateral aspect. The tubercle of the scaphoid attaches the 1. Insertion of Abductor pollicis brevis and 2. Lateral end of the Flexor retinaculum

Palpation—the scaphoid can be easily palpated on the floor of the anatomical snuff box.

Articulations of the scaphoid

Proximally – radius

Distally- trapezium and trapezoid

Medially- lunate and head of capitate

Clinical notes on scaphoid

The scaphoid is the most commonly fractured bone of the carpus. Usually the neck of the scaphoid bone is fractured. Following a fracture of the scaphoid bone, the area of tenderness is located in the anatomical snuff box. The fractured scaphoid can be slow to heal because of the limited circulation to the bone. It receives its blood supply primarily from lateral and distal branches of the radial artery. Although it is relatively difficult to break, it is the most commonly fractured bone in the carpus, particularly because of its unique anatomy and position within the wrist. Approximately 60% of carpal fractures are scaphoid fractures.

In about 10% of individuals, the scaphoid bone has only blood supply from the radial artery, which enters through the distal portion of the bone to supply the proximal portion. When a fracture occurs across the waist of the scaphoid, the proximal part of the scaphoid undergoes **avascular necrosis**.

A condition called scapholunate instability can occur when the scapholunate ligament (connecting the scaphoid to the lunate bone) is disrupted.

Fractures of the scaphoid must be recognized and treated quickly, because prompt treatment is the key to proper healing. Delays may complicate healing. Even rapidly immobilized fractures may require surgical treatment, including use of the Herbert screw to bind the two halves together.

Other carpal bones

The **lunate bone is the most commonly displaced carpal bone**.

The **lunate** is a moon-shaped bone between scaphoid and triquetral bones; it also articulates with the distal end of the radius, capitate and hamate bones.

The lunate may be dislocated due to a fall on the dorsiflexed the wrist. Dislocated lunate may cause **carpal tunnel syndrome. Dislocated lunate can result in avascular necrosis.**

The **triquetrum** is a pyramidal bone on the ulnar side of the proximal row of carpal bones. It articulates with the articular disc of the distal radioulnar joint. It also ariculates with the pisiform, lunate, and hamate bones.

The **trapezium** is a multiangular bone on the lateral (radial) side of the distal row of the carpal bones, between the scaphoid and first metacarpal bone. It also articulates with the trapezoid. It is identified by a tubercle and a groove on the palmer surface.

The **trapezoid** is also multiangular but smaller than the trapezium bone. The trapezoid articulates with the trapezium, 2nd metacarpal, capitate and scaphoid bones

The **styloid process of the ulna** is a short, round, posterolateral protuberance of the lower end of the ulna. The vertical groove between the head and styloid process lodges extensor carpi ulnaris. The apex of the ulnar styloid process is the site of attachment of ulnar collateral ligament.

The **pisiform** is a carpal bone that functions as a **sesamoid** bone in the tendon of the **flexor carpi ulnaris muscle**. It also gives origin to the abductor digiti minimi muscle.The pisiform lies on the **palmar surface** of the triquetrum.

The **hamate** is a wedge-shaped bone on the ulnar side of the hand. It articulates with the 4th and 5th metacarpal bones. It has a distinctive hook that extends on the palmar aspect. The hook of the hamate **(hamulus)** may be fractured in **golfers**. The ulnar nerve can be palpated against the **hook of the hamate**.

The **capitate** is the **largest** of all carpal bones. It articulates with the 2nd, 3rd and 4th metacarpal bones distally. It also articulates with the carpal bones like trapezoid, scaphoid, lunate, and hamate.

The Hand and Metacarpal Bones

The five metacarpal bones form the skeleton of the hand between the carpus and phalanges. These are miniature long bones consisting of bases (proximal ends); shafts (bodies) and heads (distal ends).The heads of the metacarpal bones form the knuckles of the fist. The

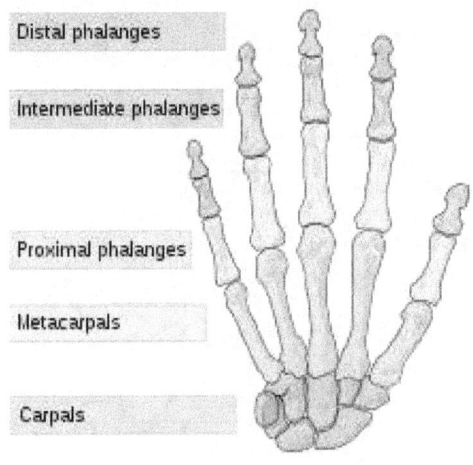

Distal phalanges

Intermediate phalanges

Proximal phalanges

Metacarpals

Carpals

proximal **bases of the metacarpals** articulate with the distal row of carpal bones.The distal **heads of the metacarpals** articulate with the proximal phalanges and form the knuckles.The **first metacarpal** is the thickest and shortest of all metacarpals.

*The first metacarpal bone receives the following muscular attachments

1. Insertion of the opponens pollicis muscle (an intrinsic muscle of the hand) along the lateral margin of the shaft.

2. Insertion of abductor pollicis longus (a deep extensor muscle of the forearm) at the base of the lateral aspect.

3. Origin of the first palmar interossei muscle (an intrinsic muscle of the hand) along the medial margin of the shaft

(Wikipedia.org; Free Encyclopedia)

Applied Anatomy: Handlebar Neuropathy

It is seen among the long distance bicycle riders.Pressure on the hook of the hamate compresses the ulnar nerve causing sensory loss along the medial side of the hand and weakness of the intrinsic muscles of the hand.

Applied Anatomy: Dermatoglyphics

Science of studying ridge patterns of the palm is called dermatoglyphics .   Simian crease (a single transverse crease) is seen among the Down syndrome patients.

Applied Anatomy: Bull Rider's Thumb

Sprain of the radial collateral ligament of the thumb. Avulsion fracture of the lateral part of the proximal phalanx of the thumb. Commonly seen in individuals who ride mechanical bulls

Applied Anatomy: Skier's Thumb

Rupture or chronic laxity of the collateral ligament of the 1st metacarpophalangeal joint and hyperabduction of the MP joint of the thumb

Each hand has 14 phalanges. There are three phalanges for each finger and two for the thumb. A phalanx has a base, shaft, and head.

Objective Questions

Q 1. Which muscle inserts to the anterior aspect of the coronoid process?

Q2. Which part of the bone (proximal and distal) the head of the radius and ulna located?

Q3. What muscle takes origin from the a. supraglenoid tubercle and b. infraglenoid tubercle of the scapula?

Q4. Which bone has a trochlea and capitulum? Name the a. proximal and b. distal row of carpal bones.

Q5. What muscles supinate the forearm and what are their innervations?

Q6. Define sesamoid bone. Name the muscles of the upper limb containing sesamoid bones.

Q7. Which of the carpal bone is the most frequently fractured?

Q8. What is the mode of blood supply of the scaphoid? Why does the head of the scaphoid undergo avascular necrosis or nonunion due to fracture of the bone?

Q 9.What muscles attaches to the first metacarpal bone? Which metacarpal bone is the thickest and shortest of all metacarpals?

Joints of the Wrist, Hand, and Fingers

Name of the joint and articulating bones	Type of joint	Movements and muscles acting on the joint	Nerve supply	Blood supply	Ligaments
Wrist joint **Articulating bones** Lower end of the Radius Scaphoid, Lunate, and Triquetral bones	Ellipsoid type of synovial joint	**Flexion**: flexor carpi radialis, flexor carpi ulnaris, and palmaris longus Assisted by flexor digitorum superficialis and flexor digitorum profundus **Extension:** Extensor carpiradialis longus, extensor	Anterior and posterior interosse ous nerves	Anterior and posterio r carpal arches	Articular capsule, palmar carpal ligaments, dorsal radiocarpal ligaments, radial collateral ligament, and ulnar collateral ligament. *Triangular

		carpi radialis brevis, and extensor carpi ulnaris Assisted by the extensors of the finger and thumb **Abduction**: abductor pollicis longus,flexor carpi radialis,extensor carpi radialis longus, and extensor carpi radialis brevis **Adduction** of the wrist is done by the simultaneous contraction of the extensor carpi ulnaris and flexor carpi ulnaris			articular fibrocartilage disc
Intercarpal joints Joints between the carpal bones	Plane type of synovial joints	Gliding movements between the carpal bones concomitantly with movements at the wrist joint	Anterior interosseous nerve Dorsal and deep branches of the ulnar nerve Posterior interosseous nerve	Dorsal and palmar carpal arches	Anterior, posterior , and interosseous ligaments
Carpometacarpal and	Plane type of	The carpometacarpal	Anterior interosse	Dorsal and	Joint

| intermetacarpal joints | synovial joint Exception: Carpometacarpal joint of the thumb is saddle type of synovial joint | joint of the thumb permits angular movements at any plane— flexion,,abduction, adduction, opposition, and circumduction Almost no movement occurs at the carpometacarpal joints of the index and middle finger, ring finger is slightly mobile, and the little finger is moderately mobile. | ous nerve Posterior interosseous nerve Dorsal and deep branches of the ulnar nerve | palmar carpal arches Deep palmar arch Metacarpal arteries | capsule Palmar and dorsal carpometacarpal and intermetacarpal ligaments |
| Metacarpophalangeal and interphalangeal joints | Metacarpophalangeal joints are condylar type of synovial joint Interphalangeal joints are hinge type of synovial joint | Metacarpophalangeal joints permit— flexion, ,abduction, and adduction Interphalangeal joints permit--- flexion and extension | Digital branches of the anterior and posterior interosseous nerves Digital branches of the ulnar nerve | Digital branches of the superficial palmar arch Digital branches of the metacarpal arteries | Fibous capsule Medial and lateral collateral ligaments |

Notes: The ulna is separated from the radiocarpal joint by a **small triangular fibrocartilage disc which extends from the distal part of the radius to the ulnar styloid process**. The ulna does not take part in the wrist joint directly. Movements of the wrist are usually associated with the movements at the midcarpal joint (between proximal and distal row of carpal bones). Abduction of the wrist is restricted to just about 15° because of the projecting styloid process.

The lateral surface of the lower end of the radius projects downwards as a styloid process. The lateral ligament of wrist joint is attached to the tip of styloid process.

Objective Question

Q. Which bones articulate to form the wrist joint?

For each type of synovial joint, select the appropriate joint type.

1. Interphalangeal joints

2. Metacarpophalangeal joint

3. Carpometacarpal joint of the thumb

4. Wrist joint

5. Intercarpal

A. Ellipsoid

B. Plane

C. Condylar

D. Hinge

E. Saddle

Wrist and hand : Anteroposterior radiograph

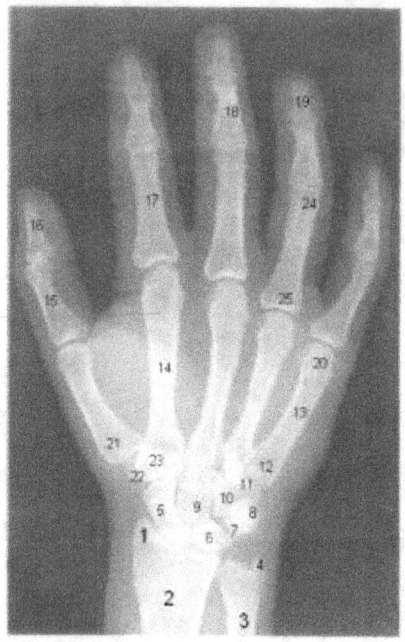

1. Radial styloid process, 2. Distal part of radius, 3. Distal part of ulna, 4. Ulnar styloid process, 5. Scaphoid, 6. Lunate, 7. Triquetrum, 8. Pisiform, 9. Capitate, 10. Hamate, 11. Hook of hamate, 12. Base of 5th metacarpal, 13. Shaft of 5th metacarpal ,14. Diaphysis of 2nd metacarpal, 15. Proximal phalanx of 1st digit, 16. Distal phalanx of 1st digit, 17. Proximal phalanx of 2nd digit, 18. Intermediate phalanx of middle finger, 19. Distal phalanx of 4th digit, 20. Head of 5th metacarpal, 21. Base of 1st metacarpal, 22. Trapezium, 23. Trapezoid, 24. Head of proximal phalanx of 4th digit, 25. Base of proximal phalanx of 4th digit (Wikipedia.org; Free Encyclopedia).

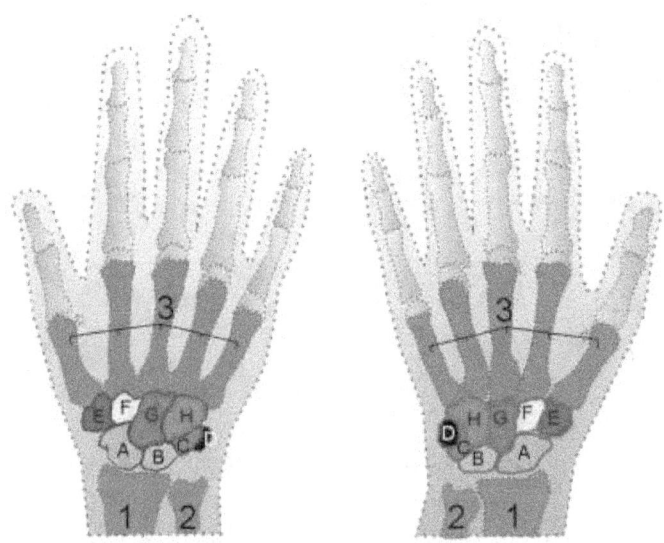

Proximal:

- A-Scaphoid
- B-Lunate
- C-Triquetrum (Triangular)
- D-Pisiform

Distal:

- E-Trapezium
- F-Trapezoid
- G-Capitate
- H-Hamate

1—indicates radius; 2—indicates ulna; 3 –indicates the middle finger

(Wikipedia.org; Free Encyclopedia)

The Shoulder and Scapular Region

The shoulder is the upper part of the superior extremity surrounding the shoulder joint.

The shoulder region has three bones:

1. The clavicle and scapula (**pectoral girdle or shoulder girdle**) and

2. The upper end of the humerus

Palpable Bony Landmarks

The spine of the scapula, vertebral and lateral borders of the scapula, and the inferior angle of the scapula.

The upper part of the scapula is covered anteriorly, laterally, and medially by the deltoid muscle.

The greater tubercle of the humerus forms the most lateral bony point of the shoulder.

The Cutaneous Innervations over the Skin of the Shoulder Region

1. The supraclavicular nerve (C3, C4) over the upper half of the deltoid muscle

2. The upper lateral cutaneous nerve of the arm (C5, C6) over the lower half of the deltoid muscle

3. The posterior rami of the upper thoracic nerves (T1 to T7) over the scapula

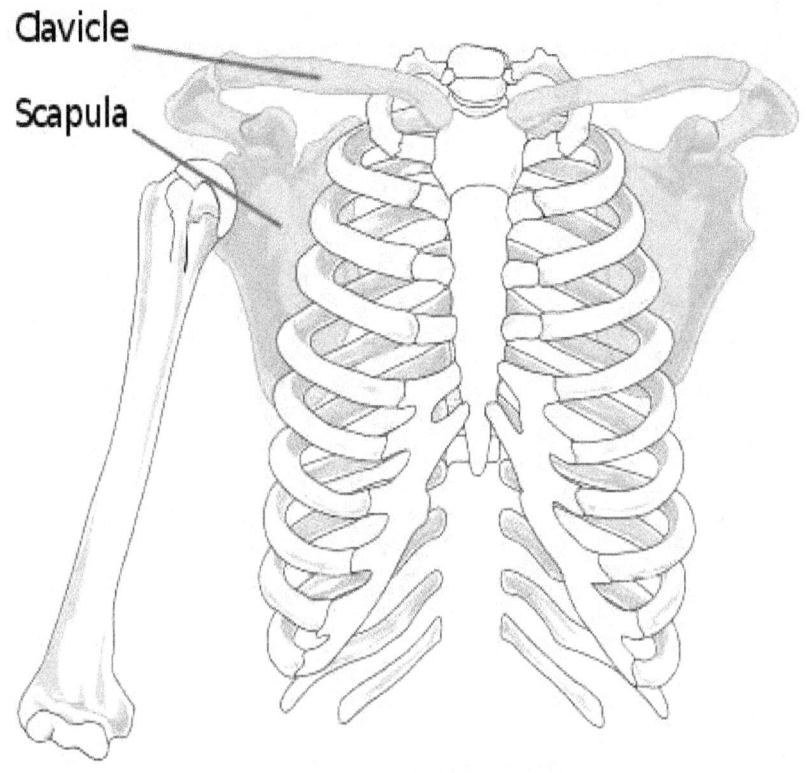

Front view

(Wikipedia.org; Free Encyclopedia)

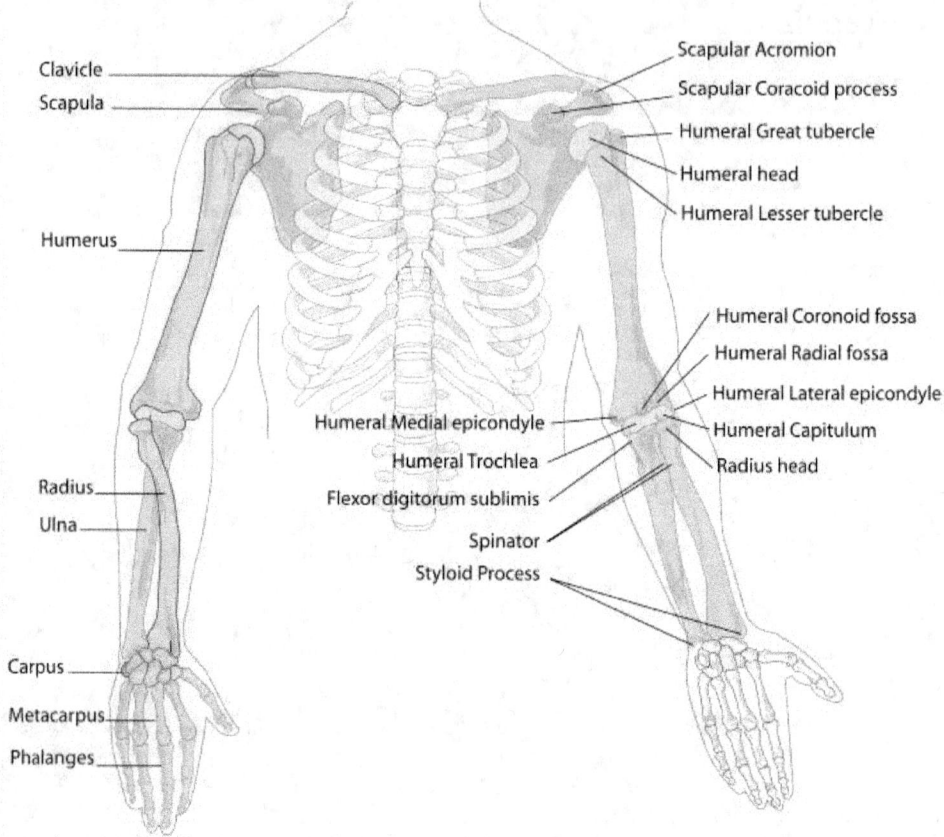

Clavicle
Scapula
Humerus
Radius
Ulna
Carpus
Metacarpus
Phalanges

Scapular Acromion
Scapular Coracoid process
Humeral Great tubercle
Humeral head
Humeral Lesser tubercle
Humeral Coronoid fossa
Humeral Radial fossa
Humeral Lateral epicondyle
Humeral Medial epicondyle
Humeral Capitulum
Humeral Trochlea
Radius head
Flexor digitorum sublimis
Spinator
Styloid Process

(Wikipedia.org; Free Encyclopedia)

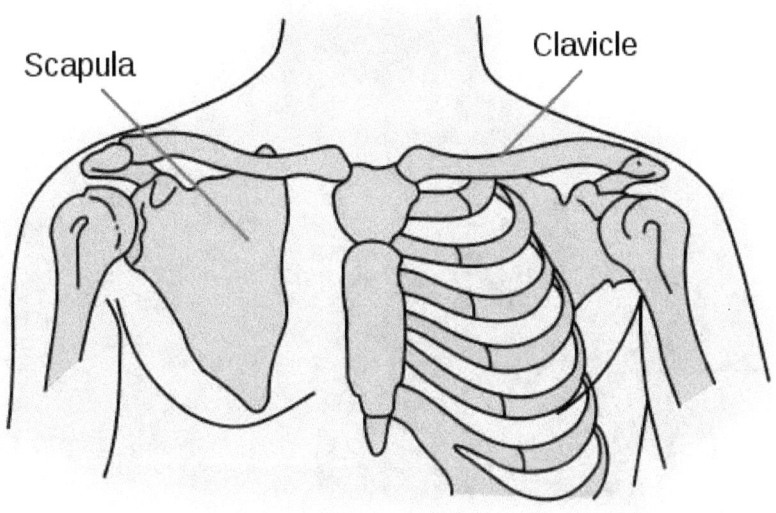

Scapula

Clavicle

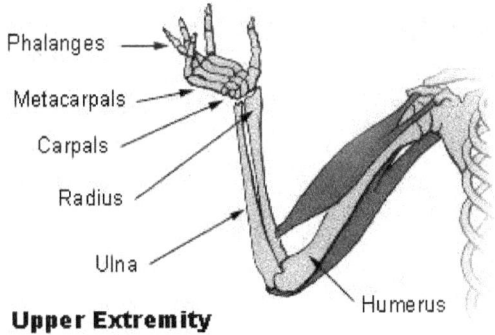

Phalanges

Metacarpals

Carpals

Radius

Ulna

Humerus

Upper Extremity

(Wikipedia.org; Free Encyclopedia)

Objective Question

Q. Which bones form shoulder girdle?

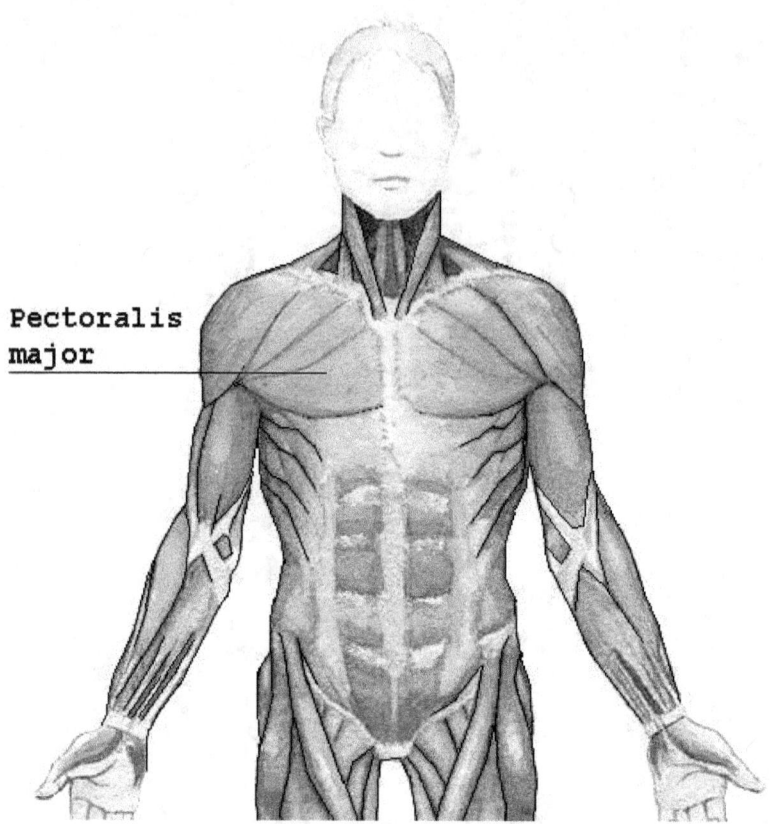

Pectoralis
major

(Wikipedia.org; Free Encyclopedia)

Spine of the Scapula

The spine of the scapula is subcutaneous. It continues from the acromion process of the scapula medially and inferiorly. The medial end of the scapular spine is called the root of the scapular spine, **located opposite to the T3 spinous process.**

The spine of the scapula divides the dorsal surface of the scapula into supraspinous fossa and infraspinous fossa.

The notch connecting the supraspinous and infraspinous fossae (**spinoglenoid notch**). The suprascapular artery and the suprascapular nerve pass through the spinoglenoid notch to reach the undersurface of the infraspinatus muscle.

Muscle Attachments on Spine of the Scapula

1. The trapezius inserts into the upper border of the crest of the spine of the scapula.

2. The deltoid originates from the lower border of the crest of the spine of the scapula.

3. The supraspinatus originates from the upper surface of the spine of the scapula including the medial two thirds of the supraspinous fossa.

4. The infraspinatus originates from the inferior surface of the spine of the scapula including the medial two thirds of the infraspinous fossa.

5. The rhomboid minor inserts on the medial end of the spine of the scapula.

The Acromion Process of the Scapula

The acromion process extends superolaterally from the spine of the scapula. The medial aspect of the distal end of the acromion process articulates with the lateral end of the clavicle. The **acromion angle** is formed by the union of the lateral and posterior border of the acromion process.

Muscle Attachments on the Acromion Process

1. The trapezius inserts along the medial border of the acromion process.

2. The deltoid originates from the lateral border of the acromion process.

The Coracoid Process of the Scapula

This is a hook like process of the scapula. It projects **anterolaterally superior to the supraglenoid tubercle of the scapula and inferior to the lateral end of the clavicle**. The **superior transverse scapular notch** lies medial to the root of the coracoid process.

Muscle Attachment on the Coracoid Process of the Scapula

1. Two muscles (short head of biceps brachii and coracobrachialis) take origin from the tip of the coracoid process.

2. The pectoralis minor inserts into the medial and upper aspect of the coracoid process.

Medial (vertebral) Border of the Scapula

The medial border of the scapula is thin and it extends from the superior angle to the inferior angle.

Muscles attaching along the **dorsal aspect** of the medial border of the scapula from above downwards:

1. The levator scapulae **inserts into the** medial border from the superior angle up to the root of the spine of the scapula.

2. The rhomboid minor **inserts into the** medial border opposite the root of the spine of the scapula

3. The **rhomboid major inserts** from the root of the spine of the scapula to the inferior angle of the scapula.

The serratus anterior muscle attaches the entire medial border of the **costal surface** of the scapula: One digitation from the superior angle to the root of the spine, two digitations to the medial border below the root of the spine, and five digitations to the inferior angle of the scapula.

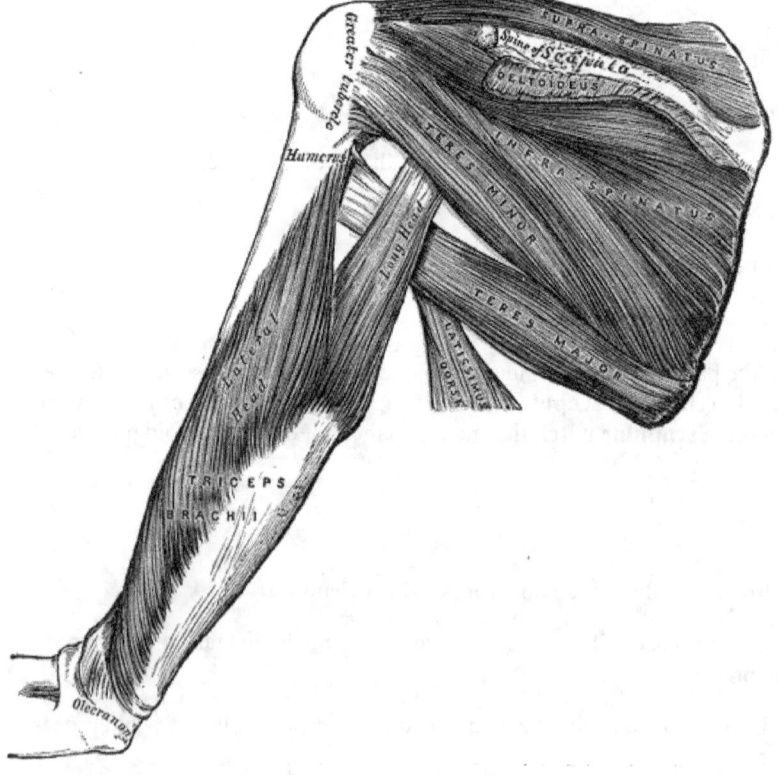

(Wikipedia.org; Free Encyclopedia)

Muscles of the Scapular Region

Muscle	Origin	Insertion	Nerve Supply	Action
Trapezius	Superior nuchal line, external occipital protuberance, ligamentum nuchae, and spinous processes of 7th cervical and all thoracic vertebrae	Superior border of the crest of the spine of the scapula, inner border of the acromion, posterior border of the lateral one third of the clavicle	Motor—Spinal root of the accessory nerve(CN XI) Sensory(pain and proprioception) C3, C4 spinal nerves	Elevates scapula during abduction of the humerus above 90°, middle fibers retracts scapula, and lower fibers depresses scapula. The upper and lower fibers, acting together, upwardly rotates the scapula (turn the glenoid cavity upwards).
Deltoid	Anterior surface of the lateral one third of the clavicle, Outer border of the acromion, and inferior border of the crest of the spine of the scapula	Deltoid tuberosity of the humerus	Axillary nerve(**C5**,C6)	Anterior fibers flexes, middle fibers abducts, and the posterior fibers extends the arm
Supraspinatus	Supraspinous fossa of the scapula	Superior facet on the greater tubercle of the humerus	Suprascapular nerve(C4,**C5**,C6)	Abducts arm first 15 Strengthens the shoulder joint by acting with other muscles of the rotator cuff

Infraspinatus	Infraspinous fossa of the scapula	Middle facet of the greater tubercle of the humerus	Suprascapular nerve(**C5**,C6)	Laterally rotates arm and stabilize the shoulder joint acting along with other muscles of the rotator cuff
Subscapularis	Subscapular fossa	Lesser tubercle of the hunerus	Upper and lower subscapular nerve(C5,**C6**,C7)	Stabilizes shoulder joint. Rotates the arm medially
Latissimus dorsi	Posterior one third of the iliac crest Spinous processes of T7 to T12 Inferior angle of the scapula and ribs 9-12	Floor of bicipital groove of humerus	Thoracodorsal nerve(**C6,C7**,C8)	Extends, adducts, and medially rotates humerus; raises body toward arms during climbing
Teres major	Oval area on the posterior surface of the lower part of lateral border of the scapula over the inferior angle	Medial lip of the intertubercular sulcus of the humerus	Lower subscapular nerve	Extends, adducts and medially rotates arm
Teres minor	Upper part of the dorsal surface of the latetral border of the scapula	Inferior facet on the posterior surface of the greater tubercle of the humerus	Axillary nerve(C5,C6)	Laterally rotates arm and stabilizes the shoulder joint
Levator scapulae	Transverse process of C1 –C4 vertebrae	Posterior surface of the upper part of the vertebral border of the scapula	Dorsal scapular nerve (C5). Anterior rami of C3 and C4 spinal nerve	Elevates scapula

Rhomboid minor	Lower part of the ligamentum nuchae and spine of C7—T1	Posterior surface of the medial border of scapula at the root of the spine of the scapula	Dorsal scapular nerve (C4,C5)	Retracts and fixes scapula by rotating and depressing the glenoid cavity
Rhomboid major	Spines of T2 to T5 and intervening supraspinous ligament	Posterior surface of the medial border of the scapula from the spine to the inferior angle	Dorsal scapular nerve (C4,**C5**)	Retracts and fixes scapula by rotating and depressing the glenoid cavity

*Injury to the spinal accessory (CN XI)** nerve primarily would affect the upward rotation and retraction of the scapula due to paralysis of the trapezius muscle. The sternocleidomastoid will be weak as evidenced by weakness in turning the head to the opposite side against resistance.

Objective question

Q. Which muscles are innervated by the spinal accessory nerve? What movements will be affected due to injury to the spinal accessory nerve?

Matching Question: For each muscle, match the most appropriate nerve.

 A. Latissimus dorsi

B. Teres major

C. Levator scapula

D. Teres minor

1. Dorsal scapular nerve

2. Lower subscapular nerve

3. Axillary nerve

4. Thoracodorsal nerve

Note. Loss of function of the supraspinatus muscle leads to inability to initiate abduction of the arm at the shoulder joint.

The deltoid muscle forms the **rounded contour** of the shoulder. The rounded contour is lost due to shoulder dislocation and by damage to the axillary nerve.

Structures under the Deltoid.

Bones

1. The upper part of the humerus

2. The coracoid process of the scapula

Muscles

Origin:

1. Short head of the biceps brachii and coracobrahialis from the tip of the coracoids process

2. Long head of the biceps brachii from the supraglenoid tubercle of the scapula

3. Long head of the triceps brachii from the infraglenoid tubercle of the scapula

4. Lateral head of the triceps brachii from the posterosuperior part of the humerus

Insertion:

1. Pectoralis major, teres major and latissimus dorsi on the intertubercular sulcus of the humerus

2. Subscapularis on lesser tubercle of humerus

3. Supraspinatus, infraspinatus, and teres minor on the greater tubercle of the humerus

4. Pectoralis minor on the coracoids process of the scapula

Clinical testing of the deltoid muscle-Deltoid is seen and felt to contract when the arm is abducted against resistance.

Rotator cuff muscles are as follows:

1. Supraspinatus

2. Infraspinatus

3. Teres minor

4. Subscapularis

MNEMONICS: **SITS** muscles

All the muscles of the rotator cuff are located in the posterior scapular regin **except** the subscapularis.Testing abduction and medial and lateral rotation of the humerus at the shoulder joint tests motor function mainly of C5 and C6 segment of the spinal cord.

Rotator cuff muscles make a musculotendinous ring around the shoulder joint, connect the scapula to the humerus and reinforce the fibrous capsule of the shoulder joint. Much of the **support for the shoulder joint** is given by the rotator cuff muscles and not ligaments. Dislocation of the humerus most often happens inferiorly because this region has the smallest amount of support.

The Tendon of the Supraspinatus

The tendon of the supraspinatus passes underneath the acromion and acromioclavicular ligament. The subacromial bursa separates the supraspinatus tendon from the acromion process. The tendon then passes over the shoulder joint and inserts on the superior facet of the greater tubercle. The supraspinatus tendon is relatively avascular. The tendon is susceptible to partial or full thickness tears as the age advances. Repeated trauma makes the tendon inflamed called **supraspinatus tendinitis**. There may be **calcium deposition** in the damaged supraspinatus tendon. Movement of the supraspinatus may be extremely painful.

Rotator Cuff Syndrome

The supraspinatus tendon may be involved in rotator cuff impingement and tendinopathy. Inflammation of the supraspinatus tendon, excessive fluid in the subacromial bursa, or subacromial bony spurs may produce significant impingement of the shoulder joint **especially in abduction**. The rotator cuff syndrome may be treated by steroid or local anesthetic injections.

Note: The supraspinatus tendon is the most frequently torn part of the rotator cuff. This injury is usual in baseball pitchers.

Subacromial Bursa

Subacromial bursa is also called subdeltoid bursa. Superiorly it is bounded by the acromion process of the scapula, coracoacromial ligament and deltoid. Inferiorly it is bounded by the supraspinatus tendon and the joint capsule of the shoulder joint. The subacromial bursa facilitates the movement of the supraspinatus tendon and the deltoid muscle. The subacromial bursa is a large bursa and it normally **does not** communicate with shoulder joint cavity. Inflammation of the subacromial bursa causes painful and restricted abduction of the shoulder joint

Synovial Bursa (e.g., subacromial bursa)

A synovial bursa is a closed bag of synovial membrane containing synovial fluid, located around the joints and tendons. Bursae regularly intervene between structures such as tendon and bone, tendon and joints, or skin and bone, and decrease the friction of one structure moving over the other.

Objective Questions

Q 1. What is a synovial bursa? What is the function of subacromial bursa?

Q 2. What is supraspinatus tendinitis?

Q 3. Which muscles form the rotator cuff?

Q 4. Which muscle is most commonly damaged in rotator cuff injuries?

Suprascapular Notch and Superior Transverse Scapular ligament

The superior border of the scapula has a suprascapular notch near the root of the coracoid process. The superior transverse scapular ligament bridges across the suprascapular notch and converts it into suprascapular foramen. The suprascapular foramen **transmits** suprascapular nerve. The suprascapular vessels pass **above** the superior transverse scapular ligament. A **lesion to the suprascapular nerve** and the suprascapular foramen results in inability to initiate abduction of the arm at the shoulder joint and to a decreased ability to rotate the arm externally.

MNEMONICS

Army marches over the bridge

Navy passes under the bridge

*Bridge—Superior transverse scapular (suprascapular) ligament

*Army---Suprascapular Artery

*Navy---Suprascapular nerve

Quadrangular Space

The quadrangular space is a passageway for the axillary nerve and posterior circumflex humeral artery from the axilla to the undersurface of the deltoid muscle.

Boundaries

Above—Inferior border of the teres minor (posterior view) and subscapularis (anterior view)

Below---Upper border of the teres major

Medially---Lateral margin of the long head of the triceps brachii

Laterally---Surgical neck of the humerus

Contents---1. Axillary nerve 2. Posterior circumflex humeral vessels

Qudrangular Space Syndrome—the quadrangular space may be decreased by hypertrophy or fibrosis of the surrounding muscles. The axillary nerve may be impinged. As a result, the deltoid and teres minor muscles become weak and non-functional.

MCQ

Which of the following arteries passes through the quadrangular space?

A. Anterior circumflex humeral artery

B. Circumflex scapular artery

C. Subscapular artery

D. Suprascapular artery

E. Posterior circumflex humeral artery

Triangular Space

Triangular space is a communication between the axilla and posterior scapular region.

Boundaries

Above---Lower border of the teres minor

Below---Upper border of the teres major

Laterally---Medial border of the long head of triceps brachii

Contents

Circumflex scapular vessels

Note: The circumflex scapular artery disrupts the origin of the teres minor, goes to the infraspinous fossa and anastomoses with the suprascapular artery.

Triangular Interval (Lower triangular space)

The triangular interval is an osseomuscular interval through which the radial nerve and profunda brachii vessels passes obliquely downwards from the medial to the posterolateral aspect of the arm.

Boundaries

Above---Lower border of the teres major

Laterally---Medial border of the shaft of the humerus

Medially---Lateral border of the long head of the triceps brachii

Contents

1. Radial nerve

2. Profunda brachii vessels

Axillary Nerve

The axillary nerve arises from the posterior cord of the brachial plexus.The axillary nerve exits the axilla through the quadrangular space in the posterior wall of the axilla. It passes around the posterior aspect of the upper part of the humerus (the surgical neck). In the surgical neck of the humerus, the axillary nerve accompanies the posterior circumflex humeral artery (a branch of the axillary artery).

The axillary nerve innervates **two muscles**—1. Deltoid and 2. Teres minor

The axillary nerve carries pain, touch, and temperature sensations from the skin of the lower part of the deltoid muscle through **superior lateral cutaneous nerve**, a branch of the axillary nerve.

Surface anatomy: The axillary nerve may be indicated as a horizontal line on the deltoid muscle, 2 cm above the midpoint between the acromion process and the middle of the humerus.

Clinical notes:

Axillary nerve may be injured by anteroinferior dislocation of the shoulder joint, injection over the axillary nerve, or by the fracture of the **surgical neck of the humerus**. As a result of axillary nerve injury the round contour of the shoulder is lost. There will be paralysis of the deltoid and teres minor muscle. The posterior circumflex humeral artery accompanying the axillary nerve may also be in jeopardy. The acromion process becomes very prominent.There is formation of depression below the acromion process. The injured person cannot abduct arm from 15°to 90°. There is anesthesia of the skin over the lower part of the deltoid muscle.

Anastomosis around the scapula

Three major arteries anastomoses in the posterior scapular region: 1. Suprascapular artery, a branch of thyrocervical trunk, 2. Deep branch of the transverse cervical artery a branch of thyrocervical trunk, and the 3. Circumflex scapular artery, a branch of subscapular artery.

Objective question

Q. What are the contents of the a. Triangular space b. Triangular interval?

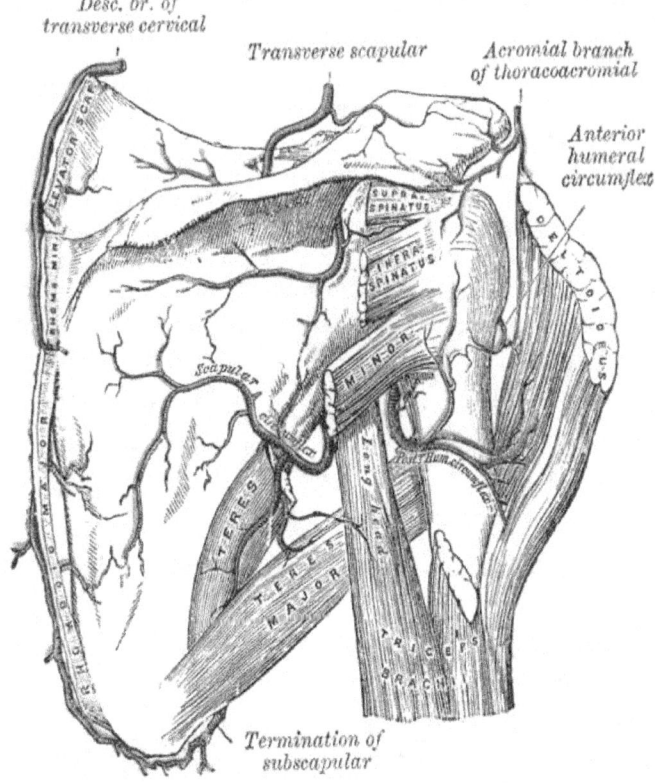

Figure. Anastomoses around the scapula

(Wikipedia.org; Free Encyclopedia)

Importance of the anastomosis around the scapula

This is an anastomosis between the first part of the subclavian artery and the third part of the axillary artery. The anastomosis provides a collateral circulation to the upper limb when the distal part of the subclavian artery or the proximal part of the axillary artery is blocked.

Subclavian artery

The **right subclavian artery** is a branch of brachiocephalic trunk. The **left subclavian artery** is a branch of arch of the aorta.

The subclavian artery is divided into **three parts** by the scalene anterior muscle.

The **transverse cervical artery** is a branch of the thyrocervical trunk.

Surface Landmarks

Scapula (shoulder blade)-The scapula is located on the posterolateral part of the upper part of the thorax. The **scapula extends** from the **2nd to 7th ribs**. The **acromion process is an anterolateral projection of the spine of the scapula, arches over the glenohumeral joint and articulates with the clavicle**. The **spine of the scapula** runs from the acromion medially and downwards to the medial border (vertebral border) of the scapula. The acromion, spine of the scapula, the medial border and the inferior angle of the scapula are **palpable structures**.

THE ARM AND THE CUBITAL FOSSA

The arm extends from the shoulder joint to the elbow joint. The humerus forms the skeleton of the arm. Medial and lateral intermuscular septa divide the arm into an anterior or flexor compartment and a posterior or extensor compartment. Structures in the front of the arm continue across the elbow joint into the cubital fossa. The arm is also called the brachium.

The artery and muscles are named accordingly, like brachial artery, brachialis, coracobrachialis, biceps brachii, and triceps brachii.

Functions of the intermuscular septa:

1. Provides additional surface for the attachment of the muscle
2. Forms planes for the passage of the neurovascular structures

Septa are well defined only in the lower half of the arm and are attached to the medial and lateral supracondylar ridges. The **medial intermuscular septum is pierced** by the 1. ulnar nerve and the 2. superior ulnar collateral artery. The **lateral intermuscular septum** is pierced by the 1. radial nerve and 2. the anterior descending branch of the profunda brachii artery.

Surface Landmarks in the Front of the Arm

The **deltoid** forms the rounded contour of the shoulder. The lower part of the muscle is conical and inserts into the deltoid tuberosity of the humerus located at the middle of the lateral surface of the humerus.

The biceps brachii is the most prominent muscle in the front of the arm in anatomical position. The biceps brachii tendon is distinctly palpable in the middle of the front of the elbow band.

Arm Muscles

The arm is divided into two anterior and posterior compartments by medial and lateral intermuscular septa, extension of the deep fascia (brachial fascia). These septa provides additional surface.

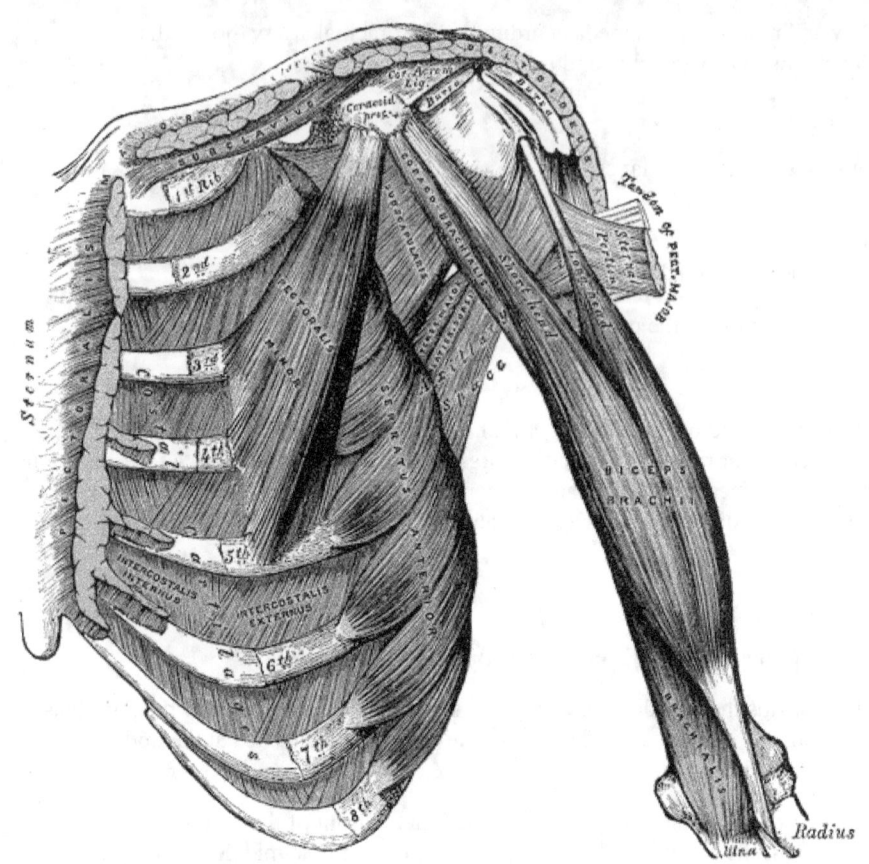

(Wikipedia.org; Free Encyclopedia)

Muscles of the arm

Muscle	Origin	Insertion	Nerve Supply	Action
Biceps brachii	Long head—supraglenoid tubercle of the scapula Short head—Tip of the coracoid process of	Posterior part of the radial tuberosity Through bicipital aponeurosis to the deep fascia of the	Musculocutaneous nerve (C5,C6)	Flexion and supination of the forearm. Flexion of the shoulder joint. Stabilization of the shoulder joint(long head)

	the scapula	forearm		
Coracobrachialis	Tip of the coracoid process of the scapula	Medial surface of midshaft of the humerus	Musculocutaneous nerve (C5&C6)	Flexion and adduction of the shoulder joint
Brachialis	Lower half of the anterior, anterolateral and anteromedial half of the humerus	Coronoid process and ulnar tuberosity	Musculocutaneous nerve (C5&C6)	Flexion of the forearm at elbow joint
Triceps brachii	Long head—infraglenoid tubercle of the scapula Lateral head—posterior surface of the humerus superior to the radial groove Medial head---posterior surface of the humerus inferior to the radial groove	Upper surface of the olecranon process of ulna	Radial nerve (C6,C7,C8)	Extension of the forearm at the elbow joint

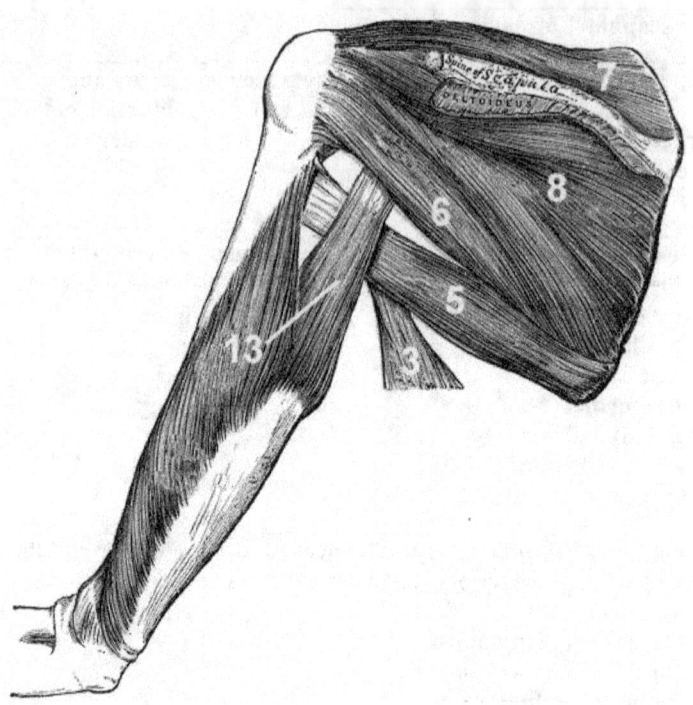

Figure: Muscles of the back of the scapula and arm. Supraspinatus (7), Infraspinatus (8), Teres major (6), Teres minor (5), Latissimus dorsi (3).Long head of Triceps brachii (13)

(Wikipedia.org; Free Encyclopedia)

Note: A "tap" on the tendon of the triceps brachii muscle tests mostly spinal cord segment **C7** (Triceps reflex). The expected finding of **triceps reflex** is visible extension of the elbow joint.

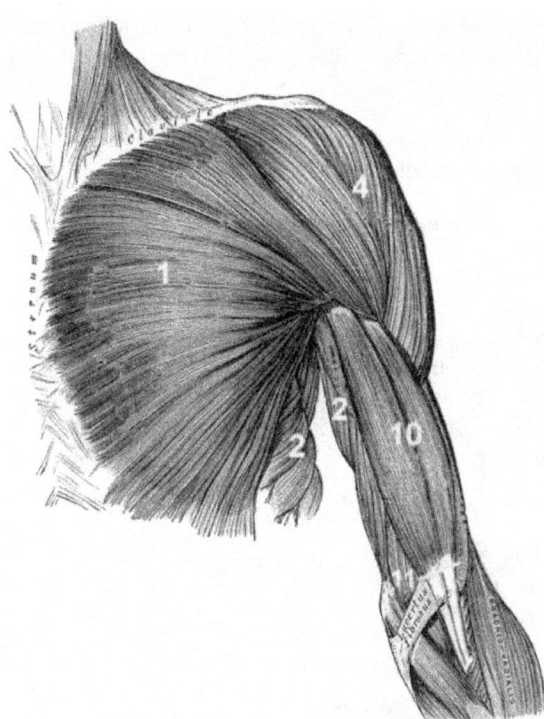

Figure: Pectoralis major (1), Serratus anterior(2), Deltoid(4), Biceps brachii(10), Tendon of biceps brachii (11) (Wikipedia.org; Free Encyclopedia)

Insertion of tendon of the biceps brachii

The tendon of the biceps brachii inserts into the **posterior part of the radial tuberosity**. It is separated from the smooth anterior part by a bursa. The tendon has a medial triangular expansion called **bicipital aponeurosis**. The bicipital aponeurosis goes down medially across the brachial artery and median nerve to blend with the deep fascia (antebrachial fascia) over the origins of the flexor muscles of the forearm and indirectly to the subcutaneous border of the ulna. The median cubital vein passes over the bicipital aponeurosis.

The **bicipital aponeurosis** affords protection for the brachial artery and the median nerve. It decreases the pressure of the biceps tendon on the radial tuberosity during pronation and supination of the forearm.

Clinical notes

Shoulder pain and long head of biceps brachii

The long head of the biceps brachii may be dislocated from the intertubercular sulcus and may cause shoulder pain. Shoulder pain is also possible with an inflamed long head of biceps brachii.

The **biceps reflex** is a deep tendon reflex. A normal biceps reflex (involuntary contraction of the biceps) confirms the integrity of the musculocutaneous nerve (C5, **C6**).

Rupture of the Tendon of the Long Head of the Biceps Brachii

The long head of the biceps brachii tendon may rupture. Rupture of the tendon commonly results from wear and tear of a sore tendon as it moves repeatedly in the intertubercular groove of the humerus. Typically the tendon is torn from the supraglenoid tubercle. Rupture of the biceps brachii tendon is seen among weight lifters, swimmers and baseball pitchers. This rupture has relatively small effect on the upper limb but it does produce a typical deformity on flexing the elbow. There is a clear-cut bulge of the muscle belly as its unstrained fibers contract—the **'Popeye' sign**.

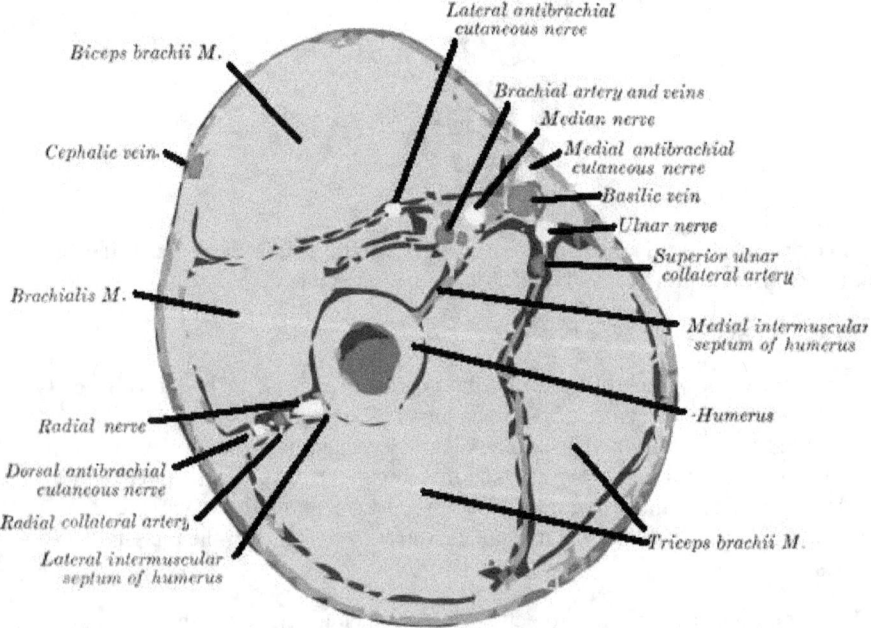

Figure: Transverse section through the mid arm (Wikipedia.org; Free Encyclopedia).

Brachial Artery

The brachial artery is the **continuation of the axillary artery** and goes from the inferior border of insertion of **the teres major muscle to the cubital fossa.** It descends medial to the biceps brachii and terminates distal to the elbow joint opposite the neck of the radius into radial and ulnar arteries.

The stethoscope bell is placed on the lower part of the brachial artery to measure the blood pressure.

The brachial pulse can be palpated immediately medial to the tendon of the biceps brachii muscle.

The brachial artery can be compressed against the humerus at the middle of the arm to stop bleeding

Branches of the Brachial Artery

1. Deep brachial artery (Arteria profunda brachii) originates near the origin of the brachial artery

2. Superior ulnar collateral artery (originates near the middle of the arm)

3. Inferior ulnar collateral artery (originates 5 cm. above the medial epicondyle of the humerus)

4. Radial artery

5. Ulnar artery

The **superior ulnar collateral artery** accompanies the ulnar nerve posterior to the medial epicondyle of the humerus. It anastomoses with the posterior ulnar recurrent artery and inferior ulnar collateral artery, participating in the anastomoses around the elbow joint.

The **inferior ulnar collateral artery** passes anterior to the medial epicondyle of the humerus and anastomoses with the anterior ulnar recurrent artery and superior ulnar collateral artery.

**Figure:
Anastomosis
around the
elbow joint.**
(Wikipedia.org;
Free
Encyclopedia)

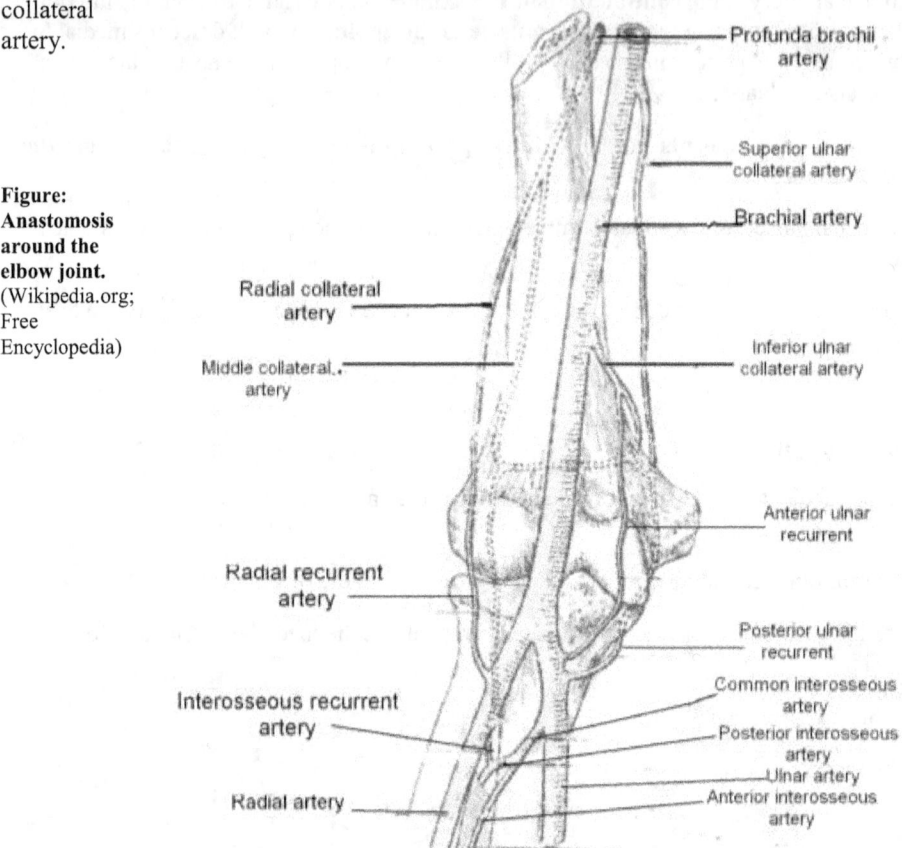

Profunda brachii artery

Superior ulnar collateral artery

Brachial artery

Radial collateral artery

Inferior ulnar collateral artery

Middle collateral artery

Anterior ulnar recurrent

Radial recurrent artery

Posterior ulnar recurrent

Common interosseous artery

Interosseous recurrent artery

Posterior interosseous artery

Ulnar artery

Anterior interosseous artery

Radial artery

  Anastomosis around the elbow joint is significant. It connects the brachial artery with the radial and ulnar arteries. It supplies the ligaments and bones of the elbow joint. Occlusion of the brachial artery during flexion of the elbow joint, or putting a surgical knot on the brachial artery, will not jeopardize circulation to the forearm.

Anastomosis around the elbow joint

In front of the medial epicondyle of the humerus	Inferior ulnar collateral artery with the anterior ulnar recurrent artery
Behind the medial epicondyle of the humerus	Superior ulnar collateral artery with the posterior ulnar recurrent artery
In front of the lateral epicondyle of the humerus	Radial collateral artery with the radial recurrent artery
Behind the lateral epicondyle of the humerus	Middle collateral branch of the profunda brachii artery with the interosseous recurrent artery

Behind the lower part of the humerus	Middle collateral branch of the profunda brachii artery with the posterior branch of the inferior ulnar collateral artery

Deep artery of arm (also called deep brachial artery, arteria profunda brachii or profunda brachii artery)

This is the largest branch of the brachial artery. It originates at the uppermost part of the brachial artery. It supplies and passes into the posterior compartment of the arm.The deep artery of the arm passes through the triangular interval accompanied by the radial nerve to the spiral groove of the humerus. Then it passes posterolaterally around the shaft of the humerus. The deep artery of the arm terminates into middle and radial collateral arteries that participate in the **anastomosis around the elbow joint**. The following are branches of the deep artery of the arm.

1. Middle collateral (posterior descending) branch

2. Radial collateral (anterior descending) branch

3. Ascending (deltoid) branch which anatomizes with the posterior circumflex humeral artery

4. Multiple muscular branches

Clinical notes:

A fracture of the humerus at midshaft may damage the deep brachial artery and radial nerve as they travel together on the posterior aspect of the humerus in the radial groove.

Radial Nerve in the Arm

The radial nerve begins from the posterior cord of the brachial plexus. It enters the arm by crossing the inferior border of the teres major. In the arm the radial nerve is posterior to the brachial artery and enters the posterior compartment of the arm accompanied by the profunda brachii artery.

Damage to the Radial Nerve in the Arm

Damage to the radial nerve above the origin of the triceps brachii muscle (e.g., pressure from long crutch-"crutch palsy") results in paralysis of the 1. Triceps brachii 2. Brachioradialis 3. Supinator and all the extensor muscles of the forearm, wrist and fingers. In addition to muscular paralysis there will be loss of sensation in areas of skin (back of the lower part of the arm, forearm and dorsum of the hand) supplied by the radial nerve.

Injury to the radial nerve in the radial groove (middle of the shaft of the humerus) results in partial paralysis of the triceps brachii (weakness triceps brachii muscle because the medial head is affected only).**The profunda brachii artery accompanying the radial nerve** in the radial groove is often affected.

 Damage to the radial nerve in any part of the arm causes **wrist drop, finger drop, inability to supinate when the elbow is extended, loss of sensation on the back of the forearm and dorsolateral surface of the hand**. A patient can not extend the wrist and the fingers at the metacarpophalangeal joints. The wrist takes a partially flexed position due to unopposed actions of the flexor muscles.

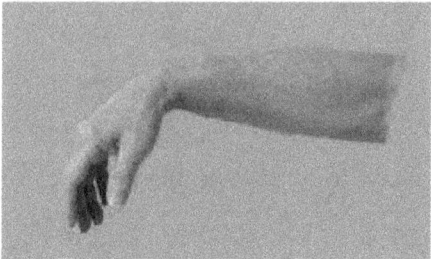

Figure: Wrist drop (Wikipedia.org; Free Encyclopedia)

Saturday Night Palsy—the radial nerve undergoes ischemic damage due to compression of the nerve against the humerus. This occurs if the arm is rested on a hard edge such as the back of the chair. There is weakness of the wrist and finger extensors and loss of brachioradialis reflex.

Wrist and finger drop may also be caused by 1. Lead poisoning 2. Multiple sclerosis 3. Guillain-Barre syndrome and 4.Myasthenia gravis

Musculocutaneous Nerve in the Arm

The musculocutaneous nerve originates from the lateral cord of the brachial plexus and contains nerve fibers from spinal cord segments **C5, C6, and C7**. It enters the arm by **piercing through the coracobrachialis** muscle. It descends obliquely through the arm in the plane between the biceps brachii and the brachialis muscles. The musulocutaneous nerve provides **motor innervations** to the 1. Coracobrachialis 2. Biceps brachii 3.

Brachialis (**the muscles of the anterior compartment of the arm**). At the lower part of the arm, it emerges lateral to the biceps brachii tendon at the elbow, penetrate deep fascia, and **continues as the lateral antibrachial cutaneous nerve (lateral cutaneous nerve of the forearm)** to provide **sensory innervations to skin on the lateral surface of the forearm** from the elbow to the wrist.

The musculocutaneous nerve provides articular innervations to the elbow joint (Hiltons law) through its branches to the brachialis muscle.

Damage to the Musculocutaneous Nerve

Damage to the musculocutaneous nerve in the axilla and arm is **uncommon** due to its shielded position. Damage to the musculocutaneous nerve causes paralysis of coracobrachialis, biceps brachii, brachialis muscles and loss of cutaneous sensation from the lateral aspect of the forearm.

Flexion of the elbow and supination of forearm is weakened but not lost. Weak flexion and supination are produced by the brachioradialis muscle (innervated by the radial nerve).

MCQ

Following a road traffic accident, a 43 year-old man developed weakness of flexion and supination of the right forearm and loss of sensation along the lateral aspect of the right forearm. Which of the following nerves has most likely been injured?

A. Axillary nerve

B. Median nerve

C. Radial nerve

D. Musculocutaneous nerve

Median Nerve in the Arm

The median nerve originates from the lateral and medial cords of the brachial plexus, enters the anterior aspect of the arm from the axilla at the inferior margin of the teres major muscle. It passes vertically downwards **along with the brachial artery** and crosses it laterally to medially. The median nerve **has no branches** in the axilla or in the arm. Occasionally a branch to the pronator teres arises from the median nerve immediately proximal to the elbow joint. It supplies articular branches to the elbow joint.

Objective Question

Q. Which nerve accompanies the brachial artery in the arm?

Ulnar Nerve in the Arm

The ulnar nerve arises in the axilla from the medial cord of the brachial plexus. It enters the arm at the insertion of the teres major. It passes medial to the brachial artery. At the middle of the arm it pierces the medial intramuscular septum with the superior ulnar collateral artery. The ulnar nerve descends between the intermuscular septum and the medial head of the triceps brachii.It passes posterior to the medial epicondyle and medial to the olecranon to enter the forearm. It is palpable at this level and is vulnerable to injury. The ulnar nerve has **no branches** in the arm but it provides **articular** branches to the elbow joint.

The ulnar nerve can be irritated at the medial epicondyle and olecranon process leading to a **"pins and needles"** sensation on the medial side of the hand. That is why they are called **funny bone or crazy bone**.

Note: Ulnar nerve is thickened in **Leprosy**.

Cubital fossa (antebrachial fossa)

The cubital fossa is a **triangular depression** on the anterior surface of the upper part of the forearm.

Boundaries:

Above (base)—an imaginary horizontal line between the medial and lateral epicondyles of the humerus

Apex of the cubital fossa is formed by the overlapping of the pronator teres by the brachioradiaslis

Below and medially—lateral margin of the pronator teres

Below and laterally--- medial margin of the brachioradialis

Floor---Bracihalis and supinator

Roof--- skin, superficial fascia, deep fascia (antebrachial fascia), and bicipital aponeurosis

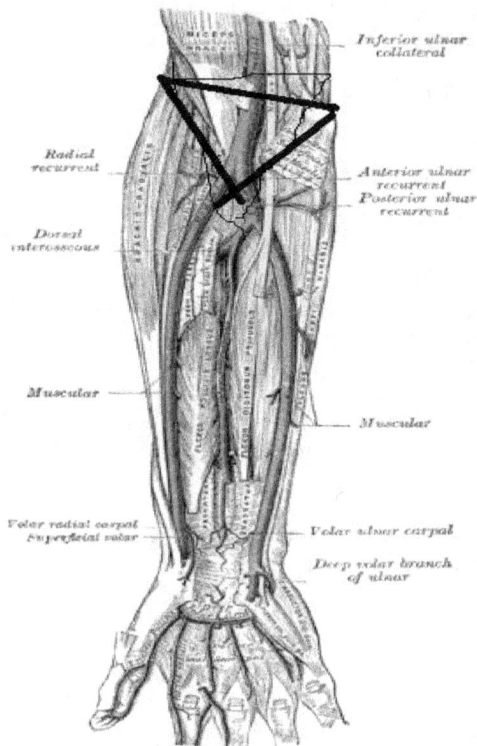

Figure. The triangular area represents the cubital fossa (Wikipedia.org; Free Encyclopedia)

Major Contents of the Cubital Fossa

1. Biceps brachii tendon

2. Terminal part of brachial artery and accompanying veins

3. Median nerve

4. Beginning of the radial and ulnar arteries

5. Radial nerve with radial collateral arteries

Notes:

A "tap" on the tendon of the biceps brachii muscle tests spinal cord segment C5 and **C6** (**Biceps Reflex**).

The brachial artery bifurcates into the radial and ulnar arteries in the cubital fossa.At the base of the cubial fossa; the brachial artery lies medial to the biceps brachii tendon.

The stethoscope bell is placed on the brachial artery to take blood pressure.

The radial nerve passes beneath the medial edge of brachioradialis (which forms the lateral Boundaries of the cubital fossa) and divides into superficial and deep branches.

The superficial branch of the radial nerve is a sensory nerve and it gets into the forearm deep to the brachioradialis muscle.

A lesion on the superficial branch of the radial nerve results in the loss of cutaneous innervations over the lateral side of the dorsum of the hand and over the thenar eminence.

The radial nerve does not innervate any of the intrinsic muscles in the hand. An injury of the superficial branch of the radial nerve results in loss of cutaneous innervations over the lateral side of the dorsal surface of the hand and over the thinner eminence.

The deep branch of the radial nerve passes between the ulnar and humeral head of the supinator and comes out at the lower border of the supinator as posterior interosseous nerve.

The ulnar nerve is not a content of the cubital fossa.

The important structures of the **roof** are the 1. median cubital vein 2. medial cutaneous nerve of the forearm 3. lateral cutaneous nerve of the forearm and 4. Bicipital aponeurosis.

MNEUMONIC: (TAN) --- the major contents of the cubital fossa from lateral to medial are the a. biceps brachii **tendon** b.brachial **artery** and c. median **nerve**

Clinical notes

A "tap" on the **tendon of the biceps brachii** at the elbow **(Biceps reflex)** tests mainly the spinal cord segment **C6**.Visible flexion of the joint is expected in the biceps reflex.

Blood pressure measurement is extremely important part of physical examination. High blood pressure is associated with long term complications like heart failure, cerebrovascular accident, renal failure, and visual loss. The sphygmomanometer cuff is inflated around the lower half of the arm. **The stethoscope bell is placed on the brachial artery.** The pressure in the arm cuff is reduced gradually and the systolic and diastolic blood pressure is recorded.

The median cubital vein is the chosen vein for intravenous injection. Blood is often drawn from the medial cubital vein for laboratory studies and samplings. The median cubital vein is detached from the brachial artery and median nerve by the bicipital aponeurosis.

Objective Question

Q. What are the contents of the cubital fossa? How are the contents arranged, in order from medial to lateral order?

Axilla

The **axilla** (or **armpit**, **underarm**, or **outer**) is the area on the human body directly under the shoulder joint where the arm connects to the shoulder.

Boundaries of the axilla

Superiorly: by the outer border of 1st first rib, superior border of scapula, and posterior border of clavicle.

Anteriorly: by the pectoralis major, pectoralis minor and subclavius.

Posteriorly: by the subscapularis above, and teres major and latissimus dorsi below

Laterally: by the intertubercular sulcus (coracobrachialis and the short head of the biceps brachii are in the axilla.)

Medially: serratus anterior and by the ribcage

Floor/Base: by the skin (visible surface of armpit)

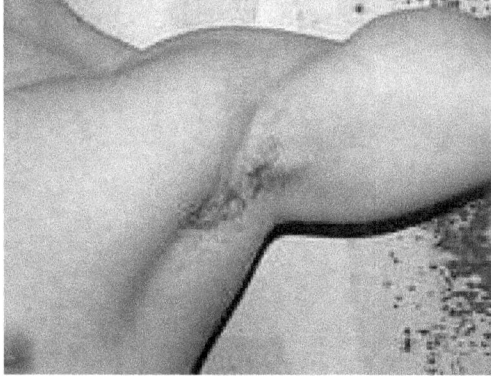

Figure: Axilla (Wikipedia.org; Free Encyclopedia)

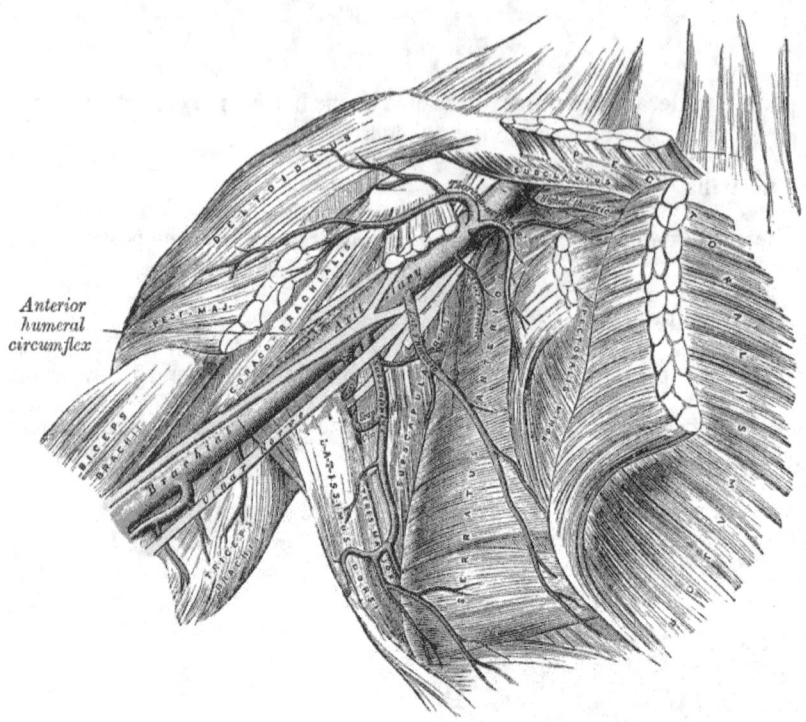

Figure: Axillary artery (Wikipedia.org; Free Encyclopedia)

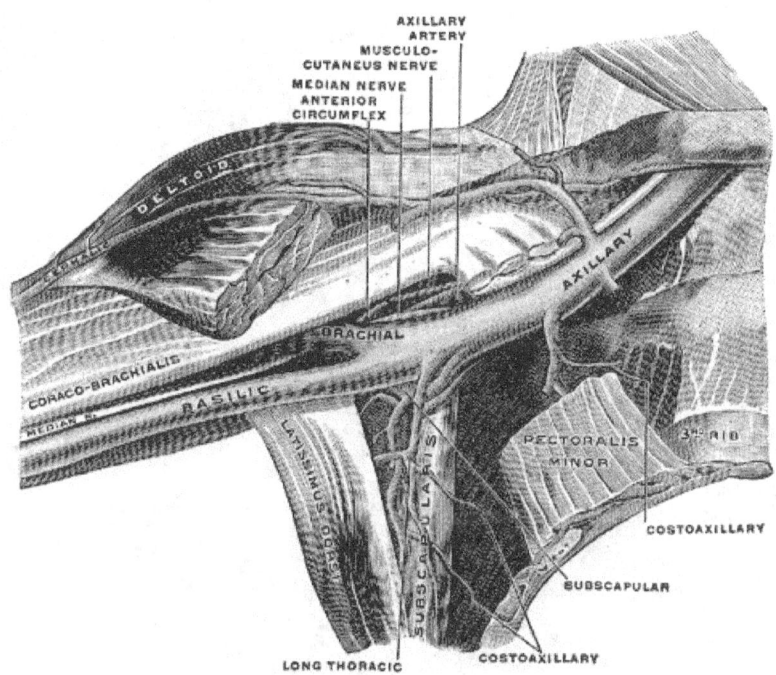

Figure: Axillary vein (Wikipedia.org; Free Encyclopedia)

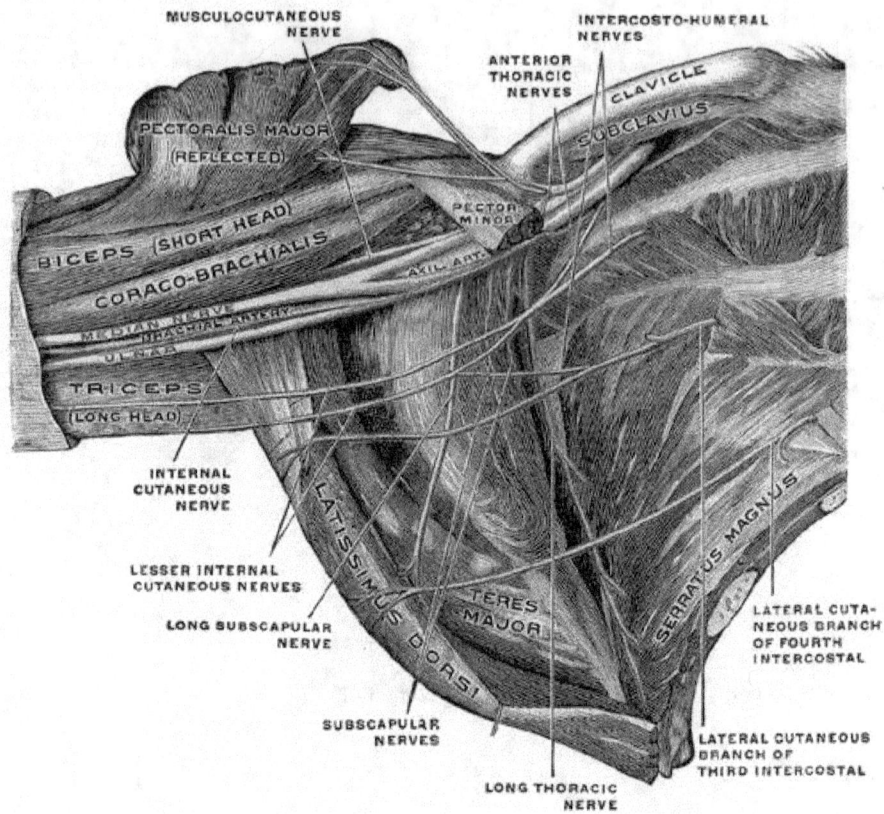

Figure: Nerves in the axilla (Wikipedia.org; Free Encyclopedia)

Contents of the Axilla

1. **Axillary artery and its branches**

2. **Axillary veins and its tributaries**

3. **Brachial plexus**

4. **Axillary lymph nodes**

5. **Intercostobrachial nerve and long thoracic nerve**

6. **Fat and loose areolar tissue**

Axillary Artery

The axillary artery is the continuation of the subclavian artery. It begins at the **outer border of the 1st rib**, passes beneath the pectoralis minor into the arm and becomes the brachial artery at the lower border of the teres major. **The axillary artery is divided into three parts by the pectoralis minor.**

1. The first part of the axillary artery is located between the lateral border of the first rib and the medial border of the pectoralis minor

The first part has one branch---the superior thoracic artery.

2. The second part of the axillary artery lies deep to the pectoralis minor and has two branches---the thoracoacromial and lateral thoracic artery

3. The third part of the axillary artery extends from the lateral border of the pectoralis minor to the inferior border of the teres major and has three branches—the subscapular artery, anterior circumflex humeral artery and posterior circumflex humeral artery.

Applied Anatomy: Aneurysm of the Axillary Artery

Abnormal dilatation of the first part of axillary artery (aneurysm) may compress the brachial plexus. There may be pain or anesthesia associated with the aneurysm of the aorta. Aneurysm may be caused by infection of the axillary artery. Repeated movement of the arm by baseball pitcher may cause aneurysm of the axillary artery.

The thoracoacromial artery is divided into four branches:

1. Acromial 2.Deltoid 3. Pectoral and 4. Clavicular.

The Thoracoacromial Artery Pierces the Clavipectoral Fascia

The lateral thoracic artery has variable origin. It usually arises from the second part of the axillary artery and descends along the lateral border of the pectoralis minor over the chest wall superficial to the serratus anterior muscle. It supplies the pectoralis major and minor, latissimus dorsi, serratus anterior, and intercostals muscles. It also supplies the lateral part of the **mammary gland** and axillary lymph nodes.

The subscapular artery gives off 1. Circumflex scapular artery and 2. thoracodorsal artery.

The anterior and posterior circumflex humeral arteries are branches of the third part of axillary artery. They surround the surgical neck of the humerus.The anterior circumflex humeral artery is smaller than the posterior circumflex humeral artery. The anterior circumflex humeral artery passes deep to the coracobrachialis and biceps brachii and supplies the shoulder joint and nearby muscles. The larger posterior circumflex humeral artery passes through the posterior wall of the axilla via the quadrangular space **accompanied by the axillary nerve** and supplies the shoulder joint and surrounding muscles.

Note:

Clinical importance of the pectoralis minor muscle

1. It divides the axillary artery into three parts.

2. It lies immediately anterior to the cords of the brachial plexus.

Objective Question

Q.What artery accompanies the axillary nerve

The Clavipectoral Fascia

The clavipectoral fascia is a part of the deep fascia that extends from the clavicle to the floor of the axilla. The clavipectoral fascia encloses two muscles—1. Subclavius and 2. Pectoralis minor

The clavipectoral fascia is pierced by the –1. Cephalic vein 2. Thoracoacromial artery 3. Lateral pectoral nerve and 4. Lymph vessels

Muscles of the Axilla

Muscle	Origin	Insertion	Nerve supply	Action
Pectoralis major (forms the anterior wall of the axilla)	**Clavicular head:** anterior surface of the medial half of the clavicle **Sternocostal head:** anterior surface of the sternum, upper six costal cartilages, and aponeurosis of external oblique muscle	Lateral lip of the intertubercula r sulcus of the humerus	Lateral and medial pectoral nerve clavicular head(C5,**C6**) sternocostal head(**C7,C8**,T1)	Flexion, adduction, and medial rotation of arm at shoulder joint
Pectoralis minor (forms the anterior wall of the axilla)	Anterior surface of the 3rd,4th, and 5th ribs near the costal	Medial border and upper surface of the coracoids	**Medial pectoral nerve(C8,T1)**	Stabilizes the scapula by pulling it down and

	cartilages	process of scapula		anteriorly
Subclavius (forms the **anterior wall** of the axilla)	**First costochondral junction**	**Inferior surface of the middle 1/3rd of clavicle**	**Nerve to subclavius** (C5,C6)	**Depresses the clavicle**
Serratus anterior(forms the **medial wall of the axilla**)	**Outer surfaces of lateral parts of 1st-8th ribs**	**Anterior surface of the medial border of the scapula**	**Long thoracic nerve(C5,C6,C7)**	**Protractio n and rotation of scapula and holds it against thoracic wall**
Subscapularis(for ms the **posterior wall of the axilla**)	**Subscapular fossa of the scapula**	Lesser tubercle of the scapula	**Upper and lower subscapular nerve(C5, C6, C7)**	**Adducts and medially rotates arm**
Teres major(forms the **posterior wall of the axilla**)	**Posterior surface of inferior angle of scapula**	**Medial lip of intertubercu lar groove of humerus**	Lower subscapular nerve(C5,C6)	**Adducts and medially rotates arm**
Latissimus dorsi (forms the **posterior wall of the axilla**)	**Iliac crest, lower 3 or 4 ribs spinous process of lower 6 thoracic vertebrae, and thoracolumbar fascia**	**Floor of intertubercu lar groove of humerus**	**Thoracodorsal nerve**	**Adducts, extends, and medially rotates humerus; elevates the body towards arm during climbing.**

Pectoralis Minor as an Important Landmark

1. The pectoralis minor lies immediately anterior to the cords of the brachial plexus.

2. The pectoralis minor lies anterior to the second part of the axillary artery.

3. The thoracoacromial artery is related to the medial or upper margin of the pectoralis minor.

4. The lateral thoracic artery is related to the lower or lateral margin of the pectoralis minor.

Note: The **subclavius** muscle acts as a **cushion** between the subclavian vessels and brachial plexus on one side and the clavicle on other side.

Nerve to the subclavius (subclavian nerve)

The nerve to the subclavius arises near the junction of the 5th and 6th cervical ventral rami. It passes posterior to the clavicle and innervates the subclavius muscle and sternoclavicular joint.

Axillary Lymph Nodes

1. Humeral (lateral) axillary lymph nodes—receive efferent lymphatic vessels from the cubital lymph nodes.

2. Apical and deltopectoral axillary lymph nodes receives lymph from the superficial lymphatic vessels accompanying the cephalic vein

Superficial abdominal lymphatic vessels superior to the transumbilical plane drain primarily to the axillary lymph nodes in the axilla.

Brachial Plexus

The **brachial plexus** is a collection of nerve fibers, running from the spine, formed by the ventral rami of the lower four cervical and first thoracic spinal nerves (C5-T1). It passes through the neck, the axilla (armpit region), and into the arm.

Functions of Brachial Plexus

The brachial plexus is responsible for cutaneous and muscular innervation of the entire upper limb, with two exceptions: the trapezius muscle innervated by the spinal accessory nerve (CN XI) and an area of skin near the axilla innervated by the intercostobrachial nerve. Lesions of the brachial plexus can lead to severe motor and sensory impairment.

Divisions and Branches of the Brachial plexus

The brachial plexus is divided into Roots, Trunks, Divisions, Cords, and Branches. There are five "terminal" branches and numerous other "pre-terminal" or "collateral" branches that leave the plexus at various points along its length.

- The five **roots** are the five ventral rami of the spinal nerves, after they have given off their segmental supply to the muscles of the neck.

- These roots merge to form three **trunks**:
    - "superior" or "upper" (<u>C5</u>-<u>C6</u>)
    - "middle" (<u>C7</u>)
    - "inferior" or "lower" (<u>C8</u>-<u>T1</u>)

- Each trunk then splits in two, to form six **divisions**:
    - anterior divisions of the upper, middle, and lower trunks
    - posterior divisions of the upper, middle, and lower trunks

- These six divisions will regroup to become the three **cords**. The cords are named by their position with respect to the <u>axillary artery</u>.
    - The <u>posterior *cord*</u> is formed from the three posterior divisions of the trunks (C5-T1)
    - The <u>lateral *cord*</u> is the anterior divisions from the upper and middle trunks (C5-C7)
    - The <u>medial *cord*</u> is simply a continuation of the anterior division of the lower trunk (C8-T1)

- The **branches** are listed below. Most branch from the cords, but a few branch (indicated in italics) directly from earlier structures. The five on the left are considered "terminal branches".

Mnemonics for remembering the order of the brachial plexus:

- **R**eal **T**exans **D**rink **C**old **B**eer
- **R**ead **T**he **D**arn **C**adaver **B**ook

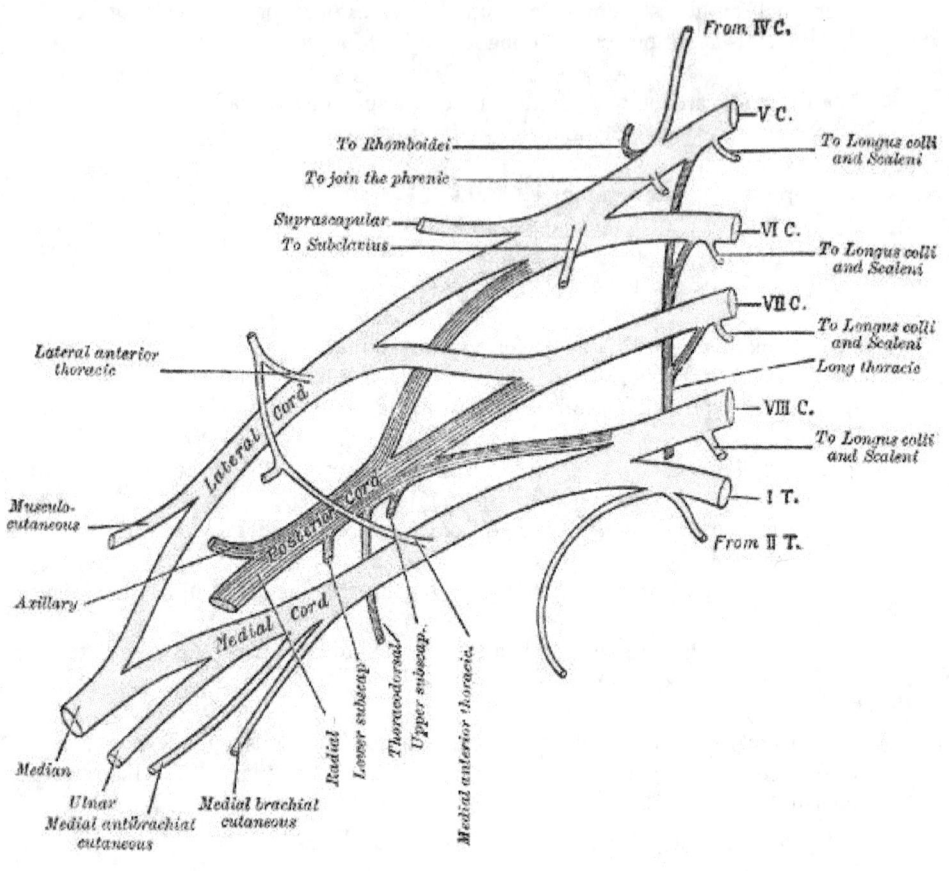

Figure: Anatomical illustration of the brachial plexus with areas of roots, trunks, divisions and cords marked (Wikipedia.org; Free Encyclopedia).

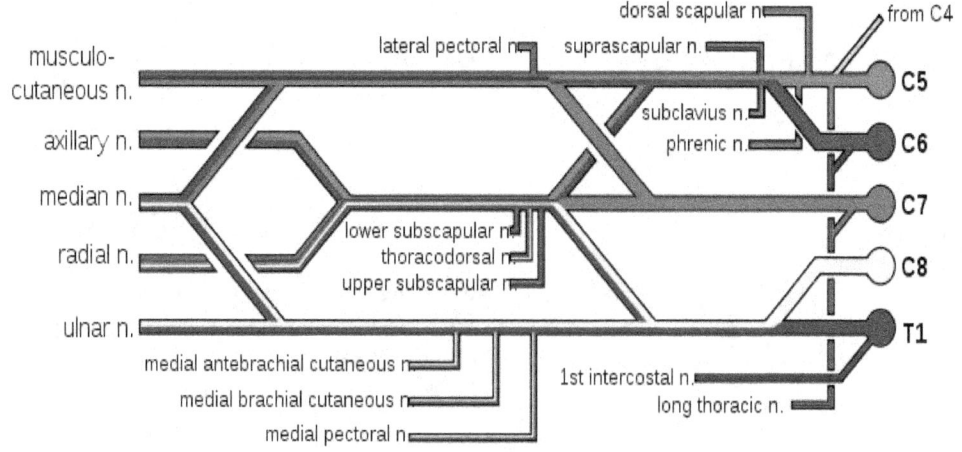

Figure: Diagrammatic representation of the brachial plexus to illustrate the contributions of each nerve root to the branches(Wikipedia.org; Free Encyclopedia)

Specific branches of the brachial plexus

From	Nerve	Root	Muscle	
Roots	Dorsal scapular nerve	C5	Rhomboid and levator scapulae	
Roots	Long thoracic nerve	C5,C6, and C7	Serratus anterior	
Upper trunk	Nerve to the subclavius	C5, C6	Subclavius muscle	
Upper trunk	Suprascapular nerve	C5, C6	Supraspinatus and Infraspinatus	
Lateral cord	Lateral pectoral nerve	C5, C6, C7	Pectoralis major (by communicating with the medial pectoral nerve)	
Lateral cord	**Musculocutaneous nerve**	C5, C6, C7	Coracobrachialis, Brachialis and Biceps brachii	becomes the lateral cutaneous nerve of the forearm
Lateral cord	**Lateral root of the median nerve**	C5, C6, C7	Fibres to the median nerve	

Posterior cord	Upper subscapular nerve	C5, C6	Subscapularis (upper part)	
Posterior cord	Thoracodorsal nerve	C6, C7, C8	Latissimus dorsi	
Posterior cord	Lower subscapular nerve	C5, C6	Subscapularis (lower part) and Teres major	
Posterior cord	**Axillary nerve**	C5, C6	Anterior branch: deltoid and a small area of overlying skin Posterior branch: teres minor and deltoid muscles	Posterior branch becomes upper lateral cutaneous nerve of the arm
Posterior cord	**Radial nerve**	C5, C6, C7, C8, T1	Triceps brachii, Supinator, Anconeus, the Extensor muscles of the forearm, and Brachioradialis	Skin of the posterior arm as the posterior cutaneous nerve of the arm
Medial cord	Medial pectoral nerve	C8, T1	Pectoralis major and Pectoralis minor	
Medial cord	**Medial root of the median nerve**	C8, T1	Fibres to the median nerve	Portions of hand not served by ulnar or radial nerves
Medial cord	Medial cutaneous nerve of the arm	C8, T1		front and medial skin of the arm
Medial cord	Medial cutaneous nerve of the forearm	C8, T1		Medial skin of the forearm
Medial cord	**Ulnar nerve**	C8, T1	Flexor carpi ulnaris, the medial 2 bellies of Flexor digitorum profundus, most of the Small muscles of the hand	the skin of the medial side of the hand and medial one and a half fingers on the palmar side and medial two and a half

Five bolded nerves are terminal nerves of the brachial plexus; then unbloded nerves are collateral nerves of the brachial plexus.

Mnemonics for remembering the branches:

- Posterior Cord Branches
  - **STAR** - Subscapular (upper and lower), Thoracodorsal, Axillary, Radial
  - **ULTRA** - Upper subscapular, Lower subscapular, Thoracodorsal, Radial, Axillary
- Lateral Cord Branches
  - **LLM "Lucy Loves Me"** - Lateral pectoral, Lateral root of the median nerve, Musculocutaneous
- Medial Cord Branches
  - **MMMUM "Most Medical Men Use Morphine"** - Medial pectoral, Medial cutaneous nerve of arm, Medial cutaneous nerve of forearm, Ulnar, Medial root of the median nerve.

Dorsal scapular nerve

The dorsal scapular nerve originates from the ventral primary rami of C4 and **C5.** It pierces the middle scalene muscle, descends deep to the levator scapulae and rhomboids, **accompanied by** the deep branch of the transverse cervical artery. It innervates the **rhomboids and occasionally the levator scapulae.**

Keys to Identify the Brachial Plexus

a. The musculocutaneous nerve pierces the coracobrachialis.

b. The median nerve begins as a Y. The two short arm of the Y are coming from the lateral cord and the medial cord of the brachial plexus.

c. The musculocutaneous nerve, median nerve and the ulnar nerve forms an M at the beginning.

Brachial Plexus Block

The brachial plexus can be numbed by injecting local anesthetic solution into or around the axillary sheath. The skin and all deep structures of the upper extremity distal to the midarm are anesthetized. Brachial plexus blocking enables surgeons to operate on the upper limb without general anesthesia.

Brachial Nerve Lesions

Erb-Duchenne Paralysis (also called waiter's tip hand)-Traumatic avulsion of nerve root contributing in the formation of **upper trunk (C5&C6).**

Traumatic avulsion of **C5 and C6 roots** can occur at birth as a result of traction on the head during delivery of the shoulder. It can also be the result of injuries caused by excessive separation of the shoulder. Erb-Duchenne paralysis is characterized by loss of shoulder abduction, lateral rotation of the shoulder and elbow flexion. The paralyzed muscles are **deltoid, biceps brachii, and brachioradialis, supraspinatus, infraspinatus, and teres minor.** The affected arm is held internally rotated at shoulder, with a pronated forearm and extended elbow. **The biceps and brachioradialis jerks are lost**, but **sensory loss is usually unremarkable, since it is confined to a small area overlying the lateral aspect of the upper limb.**

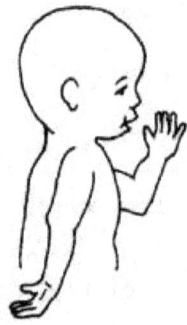

Figure: **Erb's palsy** (Wikipedia.org; Free Encyclopedia)

Treatment

Some babies recover on their own; however, some may require specialist intervention. Neonatal / pediatric neurosurgery is often required for avulsion fracture repair. Lesions may heal over time and function may return. Physiotherapeutic care is often required to regain muscle usage.

Backpacker's Palsy

The upper part of the brachial plexus injury may produce muscle spasm and a severe disability in hikers who carry heavy backpacks for long periods.

Klumpke's Paralysis

Involvement of the C8 and T1 roots causes paralysis and wasting of small muscles of the hand and of the long finger flexors and extensors. This kind of lower plexus paralysis often follows a fall that has been arrested by grasping a fixed object with one hand or may result from traction on the abducted arm. Symptoms include **claw hand**, paralysis of intrinsic hand muscles, and ulnar nerve distribution numbness. Involvement of T1 may result in Horner's syndrome, with ptosis, and miosis.

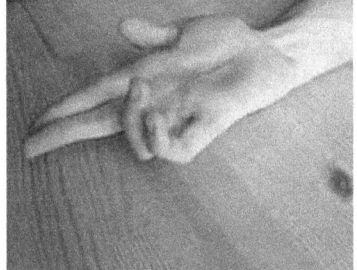

Figure: **Claw hand.**A hand imitating an ulnar claw. The metacarpophalangeal joints of the 4th and 5th fingers are extended and the interphalangeal joints of the same fingers are flexed (Wikipedia.org; Free Encyclopedia).

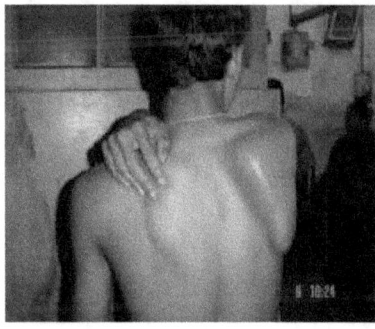

Figure: Winged scapula (Wikipedia.org; Free Encyclopedia)

The paralysis of the serratus anterior results in a **"winged scapula"** and failure to raise the arm above the horizontal. **Winging of the scapula** is demonstrated by asking the patient to push against resistance such as wall, and the arm extended at the elbow and flexed to 90° at the shoulder. Winged scapula may be demonstrated by touching the opposite scapula. The vertebral border of the scapula becomes prominent in winged scapula.

Injury to the Axillary Nerve

The axillary nerve may be injured in anterior-inferior dislocations of the shoulder joint, compression of the axilla with a crutch or fracture of the surgical neck of the humerus. Injury to the nerve results in:

1. Paralysis of the teres minor muscle and deltoid muscle resulting in loss of abduction of arm (from 15-90 degrees), weak flexion, and rotation of shoulder. Paralysis of deltoid & teres minor results in Flat shoulder deformity.
2. Loss of sensation in the skin over a small part of the lateral upper arm.

Objective Questions

1. Where the brachial plexus is located? Ventral primary rami of what spinal nerves contribute in the formation of the brachial plexus?

2. How is a spinal nerve formed? How is the middle trunk of the brachial plexus formed?

3. Which trunk of the brachial plexus provides muscular branches? The suprascapular nerve and the nerve to the subclavius are derived from which trunk of the brachial plexus?

4. Define axilla? What are the boundaries of the axilla? What are the contents of the axilla?

5. What is the course of the axillary artery? What are the branches of the axillary artery?

6. Which muscle divides the axillary artery into three parts? What are the branches of the axillary artery from each of the part of the axillary artery?

7. Which artery pierces the clavipectoral fascia?

8. Which muscle divides the subclavian artery into three parts?

9. Where is the location of the clavipectoral fascia? Which muscles are enclosed by the clavipectoral fascia? Which structures pierces the clavipectoral fascia?

10. What causes winging of the scapula? How it is best demonstrated?

Important veins of the upper limb

Axillary Vein

 The axillary vein begins at the lower border of the teres major muscle. It is a continuation of the basilic vein. The axillary vein becomes the subclavian vein at the outer border of the 1st rib.

The tributaries of the axillary vein generally follow the branches of the axillary artery. Other tributaries of the axillary veins are the brachial veins and cephalic vein.

Cephalic Vein

The cephalic vein originates at the **anatomical snuff box** from the lateral side of the **dorsal venous network** of the hand. It passes along the lateral border of the wrist and forearm to the cubital fossa. At the **cubital fossa**, the cephalic vein communicates to the basilic vein through the median cubital vein. The cephalic vein continues superiorly along the lateral border of the biceps brachii and then along the deltopectoral groove (in the **clavipectoral triangle**). It passes deep to the clavicular head of the pectoralis major and pierces the **clavipectoral fascia** and opens into the **axillary vein**.

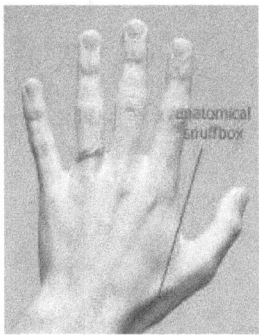

Figure: Anatomical snuff box (Wikipedia.org; Free Encyclopedia)

Basilic Vein

The basilic vein forms from the medial side of the dorsal venous network of the hand and passes into the dorsomedial aspect of the forearm. The basilica vein passes vertically in the lower half of the arm and penetrates deep fascia and lies medial to the brachial artery. It becomes the axillary vein at the lower border of the teres major muscle.

Brachial Veins

Brachial veins are paired **deep veins** accompanying the brachial artery as venae comitantes. The brachial veins begin at the elbow by union of the accompanying veins of the ulnar and radial arteries. The brachial veins open into the basilic vein and in the axillary vein.

The deep veins have numerous anastomoses with each other and with the superficial veins.

Median Cubital Vein

The median cubital vein is located in the roof of the cubital fossa. It runs diagonally from the cephalic vein to the basilic vein. The **bicipital aponeurosis separates** the median cubital vein from the median nerve and brachial artery. The median cubital vein is one of the most chosen veins for **venipuncture: for blood sampling, blood transfusion, cardiac catheterization and intravenous injection**.

It is variable in size and course. It may be vey large, in that case the distal part of the cephalic vein may be absent.

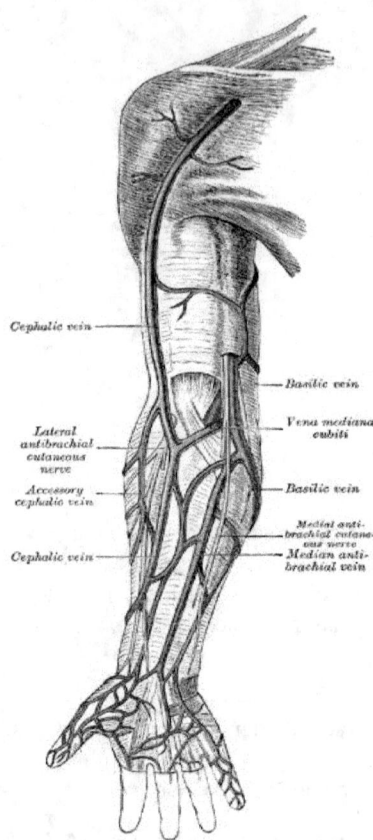

Labels on figure:
Cephalic vein
Basilic vein
Vena mediana cubiti
Lateral antibrachial cutaneous nerve
Accessory cephalic vein
Basilic vein
Medial antibrachial cutaneous nerve
Cephalic vein
Median antibrachial vein

(Wikipedia.org; Free Encyclopedia)

Objective Question

Q. What is the clinical importance of median cubital vein? What is its relationship to the cephalic vein, basilic vein, and bicipital aponeurosis?

MCQ

Q. Which of the following nerves may be punctured at venipuncture at the upper part of the cubital fossa?

A. Radial nerve

B. Ulnar nerve

C. Musculocutaneous nerve

D. Median nerve

Forearm

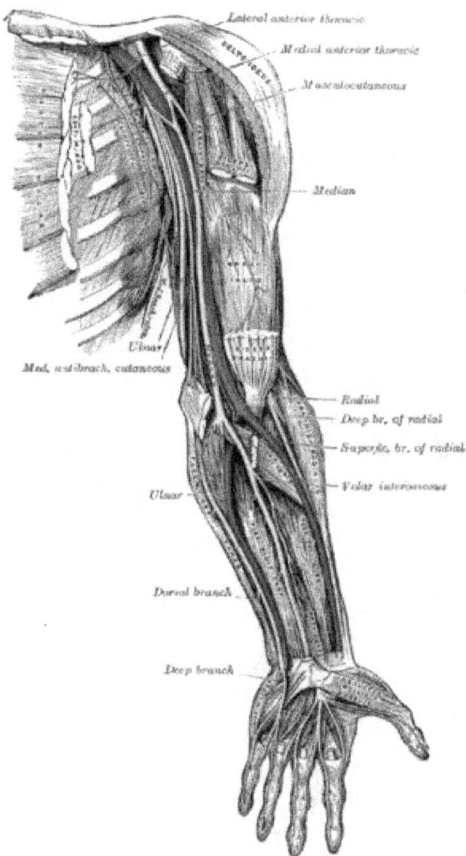

Superficial flexor muscles of the forearm (Wikipedia.org; Free Encyclopedia)

Superficial Flexor Muscles of the Forearm

Muscle	Origin	Insertion	Nerve Supply	Action
Pronator teres	Humeral head---medial epicondyle of the humerus and lower part of the	Middle of the lateral surface of the radius	Median nerve(C6,C7)	Pronates the forearm and flexes the elbow joint.

	supracondylar ridge of the humerus; Ulnar head-- from the medial side of the coronoid process of the ulna			
Flexor carpi radialis	Medial epicondyle of the humerus	Palmar surface of the base of the 2nd and 3rd metacarpal bone	Median nerve(C6,C7)	Flexes and abducts the wrist joint
Palmaris longus	Medial epicondyle of the humerus	Distal half of the flexor retinaculum and the apex of the palmar aponeurosis	Median nerve(C6,C7)	Flexes the hand and tenses the palmar fascia
Flexor carpi ulnaris	Humeral head—medial epicondyle of the humerus; Ulnar head— olecranon process and posterior border of the ulna	Pisiform bone, hamate bone, and base of the 5th metacarpal bone	Ulnar nerve(C7,C8)	Flexes and adducts the wrist joint
Flexor digitorum superficialis	Humeral head---medial epicondyle of the humerus; Ulnar head--- coronoid process of the ulna; Radial head---	Palmar surfaces of the middle phalanges of the index, middle, and ring finger	Median Nerve(C8,T1)	Flexes the proximal interphalageal joint of the index, middle,, ring, and little finger, metacarpophalangeal joints of the same fingers, and flexes the wrist joint

	Upper half of the anterior border of the radius			

Notes: The median nerve enters the forearm between the ulnar and humeral origin of the pronator teres.

The ulnar artery passes deep to the ulnar origin of the pronator teres.

The lateral margin of the pronator teres forms the medial boundary of the cubital fossa, a hollow on the upper part of the flexor aspect of the forearm.

Deep Flexor Muscles of the Forearm

Name of the muscle	Origin	Insertion	Nerve supply	Action
Flexor digitorum profundus	Shaft of the ulna, coronoid process, and interosseous membrane	Bases of the palmar surfaces of the distal phalanges of index, middle, ring and little fingers	Anterior interosseous nerve(a branch of the median nerve) for **lateral half** Ulnar nerve for the **medial half**	**Flexes the distal interphangeal joints, proximal interphalangeal joint,metacarpophalangeal joints of the index, middle,ring and little fingers** **Flexes the wrist joint**
Flexor pollicis longus	Anterior surface of the radius, medial epicondyle of the humerus, and coronoid process of the ulna	Base of the distal phalanx of thumb	Anterior interosseous nerve	**Flexes the thumb at the interphalangeal and metacarpophalangeal joint**

Pronator quadratus	Anterior surface of the distal third of the shaft of ulna	Anterior surface of the distal fourth of the shaft of radius	Anterior interosseous nerve	Pronates the forearm

Ulnar Nerve in the Forearm

The ulnar nerve comes out of the brachial plexus. It enters the anterior compartment of the forearm by passing posteriorly around the **medial epicondyle of the humerus and between the humeral and ulnar head of the flexor carpi ulnaris muscle**. It accompanies the ulnar artery between the flexor carpi ulnaris and flexor digitorum profundus muscle. In the forearm, the ulnar nerve innervates the **1. Flexor carpi ulnaris and 2. Medial half of the flexor digitorum profundus.**

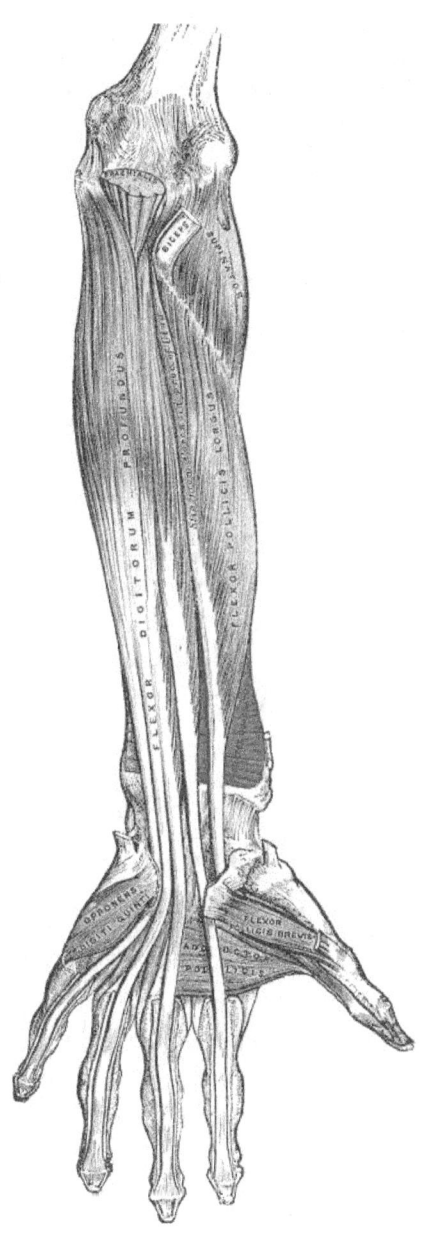 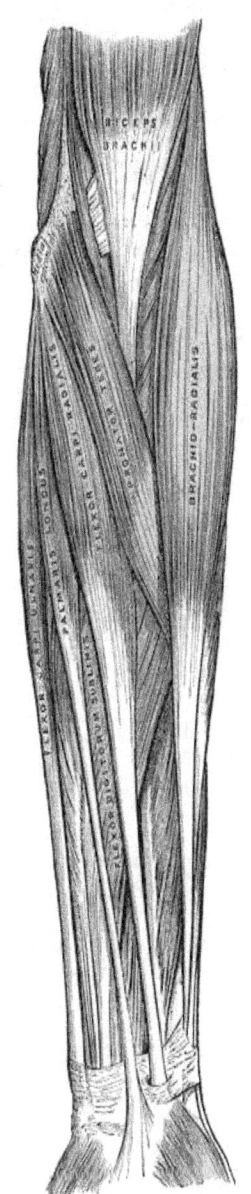

Deep flexor muscles of the forearm   superficial flexor muscle of the forearm

(Wikipedia.org; Free Encyclopedia)

Anterior Interosseous Nerve

The anterior interosseous nerve is a branch of the median nerve. The anterior interosseous nerve runs distally on the anterior aspect of the interosseous membrane, innervates the distal radioulnar joint and wrist joint. The anterior interosseous nerve is accompanied by the anterior interosseous artery, which is a branch of common interosseous artery.

Muscles Innervated by the Anterior Interosseous Nerve (a branch of median nerve)

1. Flexor pollicis longus 2. Lateral half of the flexor digitorum profundus (tendons for the index and middle finger and the 3. Pronator quadratus.

Note: All muscles in the anterior compartment of the forearm are innervated by the median nerve with the exception of the flexor carpi ulnaris and the medial half of the flexor digitorum profundus.

Ulnar artery lies lateral to the ulnar nerve.

The axillary artery lies between the lateral and medial cords of the brachial plexus.

The superior ulnar collateral artery accompanies the ulnar nerve.

The deep palmar arch lies deep to the flexor tendons on the proximal part of the metacarpals and on the interossei muscles.

The thoracodorsal artery is a branch/continuation of the subscapular artery. The subscapular artery is a branch of the third part of the axillary artery. The thoracodorsal artery accompanies the thoracodorsal nerve. The thoracodorsal nerve innervates the lattissimus dorsi.

MCQ

Q.When the **median nerve** is cut off in the elbow region, there will be **loss of** all of the following **EXCEPT:**

A. Flexion of the proximal interphalangeal joints of the index and middle fingers.

B. Flexion of the distal interphalangeal joints of the ring and little finger

C. Flexion of the proximal interphalangeal joints of the ring and little finger

D. Flexion of the wrist joint

Radial Artery in the Forearm

The radial artery is the smaller terminal division of the brachial artery in the cubital fossa.It descends downwards to the wrist and is superficial throughout its course in the forearm. It leaves the forearm by turning posterolaterally, passes over the floor of the anatomical snuff box, and reaches the palm of the hand between the two heads of the first dorsal interossei muscle and adductor pollicis muscle.

Relations of the Radial Artery in the Forearm

Anteriorly

Brachioradialis muscle in the upper part

Skin, superficial fascia, and deep fascia in the lower part

Posteriorly (from above downwards)

1. Biceps brachii tendon

2. Insertion of supinator

3. Insertion of pronator teres

4. Radial origin of flexor digitorum superficialis

5. Radial origin of flexor pollicis longus

6. Insertion of pronator quadratus

7. Lower part of the shaft of the radius

Branches of the Radial Artery in the Forearm

1. Radial recurrent artery (near the elbow joint) 2.Muscular branches to the forearm 3.Palmar carpal branches (near the wrist joint) and 4. Superficial palmar branch (near the wrist joint)

Clinical note: The radial artery is commonly palpated against the lower part of the anterior surface of the shaft of the radius to count the **pulse rate.** Here, the radial artery is located lateral to the tendon of the flexor carpi radialis muscle and medial to the abductor pollicis longus muscle.

Ulnar Artery in the Forearm

The ulnar artery is the **larger terminal branch of the brachial artery** in the cubital fossa.It departs the cubital fossa by passing deep to the pronator teres muscle. It then goes through the forearm between the flexor carpi ulnaris and flexor digitorum profundus muscle. **Branches of the ulnar artery** in the forearm include: 1. the ulnar recurrent artery with anterior and posterior branches 2.the common interosseous artery which divides into anterior and posterior interosseous arteries 3. ventral and dorsal carpal branches and 4. muscular branches

The pulse of the ulnar artery in the distal forearm is more difficult to palpate because it is placed under the anterolateral lip of the flexor carpi ulnaris muscle.

Back of the forearm

Superficial layer of muscles at the back of the forearm

Muscle	Origin	Insertion	Nerve supply	Action
Anconeus	Lateral epicondyle of the humerus	Lateral aspect of the olecranon process and the upper one fourth of the posterior surface of the ulna	Radial nerve(C6,C7,&C8)	Weak extensor of the elbow joint. Abducts the ulna during pronation
Brachioradialis	Upper 2/3rd of lateral supracondular ridge of humerus	Lateral surface of the radius just above the styloid process	Radial nerve(C5,C6,C7)	Flexes the forearm Helps in supination and pronation and keeps the forearm in midprone position
Extenso carpi radialis longus	Lower part of the lateral supracondylar ridge	Dorsal aspect of the base of the second metacarpal bone	Radial nerve(C6,C7)	Extends the wrist Abducts the wrist
Extensor carpi radialis brevis	Lateral epicondyle of humerus(common extensor origin)	Dorsal aspect of the base of the 2nd and 3rd metacarpals	Deep branch of radial nerve(C7,C8)	Extends the wrist Abducts the wrist
Extensor digitorum	Lateral epicondyle of the humerus(common extensor origin)	Extensor expansion of the index, middle, ring, and little	Posterior interosseous nerve(C7,C8)	Extends all the fingers except the thumb at the metacarpophalangeal and interphalangeal joints

		fingers		
Extensor digiti mini	Lateral epicondyle of the humerus(common extensor origin)	Extensor expansion of the little finger	Posterior interosseous nerve(C7,C8)	Extends the little fingers at the metacarpophalangeal and interphalangeal joints
Extensor carpi ulnaris	Lateral epicondyle of the humerus(common extensor origin) Posterior border of the ulna	Dorsal aspect of the base of the 5th metacarpal	Posterior interosseous nerve(C7,C8)	Extends the wrist joint Adduction of the hand

Note: The extensor carpi ulnaris tendon passes through an independent cubicle of the extensor retinaculum, in the groove between the head and styloid process of the ulna

Relations of the Brachioradialis Muscle

The tendon of the brachioradialis is crossed near its distal termination by the tendon of the abductor pollicis longus and extensor pollicis brevis. The radial artery in the lower part of the forearm is on the medial side of the brachioradialis. The brachioradialis tendon crosses the superficial branch of the radial nerve near the lower part of the forearm.

Clinical testing—The brachioradialis becomes visble and palpated when the mid-proned forearm is flexed against resistance.

Radial Nerve in the Forearm.

The radial nerve divides into a superficial and a deep branch of the radial nerve in the lateral part of the cubital fossa in front of the lateral epicondyle of the humerus and between the brachialis and brachioradialis muscles.

The superficial radial nerve is the cutaneous (sensory) nerve to the lateral part of the dorsum of the hand and anatomical snuff box. It also provides sensory innervations to the joints of the hand.

The deep branch of the radial nerve passes laterally around the radius, pierces the supinator, and reaches the posterior compartment of the forearm as the posterior interosseous nerve.

The posterior interosseous nerve passes over the posterior surface of the interosseous membrane accompanied by the posterior interosseous artery. The posterior interosseous nerve innervates most of the muscles of the back of the forearm.

Note: The **radial nerve** innervates the 1. Brachioradialis and 2. Extensor carpi radialis longus. The **deep branch of the radial nerve** innervates the 1. Extensor carpi radialis brevis and 2. Supinator.

The posterior interosseous nerve innervates the 1.Extensor digitorum 2. Extensor digiti minimi 3. Extensor carpi ulnaris 4. Extensor indicis 5. Abductor pollicis longus 6. Extensor pollicis longus and 7. Extensor pollicis brevis.

Ulnar Nerve in the Forearm

The ulnar nerve comes out of the brachial plexus. It enters the anterior compartment of the forearm by passing posteriorly around the **medial epicondyle of the humerus and between the humeral and ulnar heads of the flexor carpi ulnaris muscle**. It accompanies the ulnar artery between the flexor carpi ulnaris and flexor digitorum profundus muscles. In the forearm, the ulnar nerve innervates the **1. flexor carpi ulnaris and 2. medial half of the flexor digitorum profundus**

What is Cubital Tunnel Syndrome?

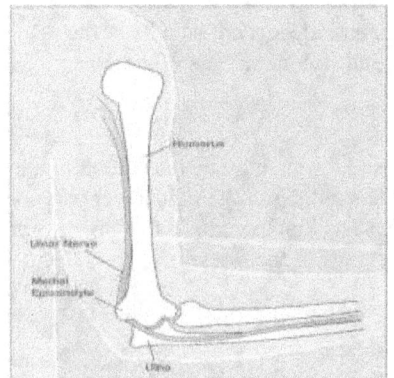

The cubital tunnel syndrome is a condition caused by increased pressure on the ulnar nerve at the elbow. There is a bump of bone on the inner portion of the elbow (medial epicondyle) under which the ulnar nerve passes. This site is commonly called the "funny bone" At this site; the ulnar nerve lies directly next to the bone and is susceptible to pressure. When the pressure on the nerve becomes great enough to disturb the way the nerve works, then numbness, tingling, and pain may be felt in the elbow, forearm, hand, and/or fingers.

Figure. Ulnar nerve in the elbow region (Wikipedia.org; Free Encyclopedia)

Signs and symptoms of the Cubital Tunnel Syndrome
Cubital tunnel syndrome symptoms typically include pain, numbness, and/or tingling. The numbness or tingling most frequently occurs in the ring and little fingers. The symptoms are generally felt when there is pressure on the nerve, such as sitting with the elbow on an arm rest, or with repetitive elbow bending and straightening. Frequently symptoms will be felt when the elbow is bent position for long period of time, such as when holding the phone, or while sleeping. Some patients may observe weakness, pinching, occasional clumsiness, and/or a tendency to drop things. In severe cases, sensation may be lost and the muscles in the hand may lose bulk and strength.

Objective Question

Q. What is the common place for measuring the pulse rate?

MCQ

A 56-year-old man developed wrist drop and weakness of grasp but normal strength of the elbow joint. There is no loss of sensation of the affected upper limb. What nerve was most likely affected?

A. Anterior interosseous nerve

B. Posterior interosseous nerve

C. Ulnar nerve

D. Musculocutaneous nerve

Radial Tunnel Syndrome

Radial tunnel syndrome is an **entrapment neuropathy of the radial nerve close to the the elbow joint**. The radial nerve may be compressed by fibrous bands of the extensor carpi radialis brevis, extensor carpi radialis longus, and supinator or by the radial recurrent artery. **Pain** on the back of the forearm is a presenting symptom of radial tunnel syndrome. Pain is exacerbated by the movement of the elbow and wrist joint. This syndrome may be **clinically tested** by flexing the patient's long finger while the patient extends the wrist and fingers. Pain is a positive finding. Usually; there is **no sensory disturbance or motor loss** in the radial tunnel syndrome.

Wartenberg's Disease (Radial sensory nerve entrapment)

The entrapment of the superficial radial nerve can occur as it emerges from underneath the edge of the brachioradialis tendon approximately 6 cm proximal to the radial styloid process. There may be a history of trauma in this part of the forearm. The symptoms are pain and paraesthesia over the lateral aspect of the dorsum of the wrist and hand.

Deep Layer of Muscles at the Back of the Forearm

Muscle	Origin	Insertion	Nerve supply	Action
Supinator	Superficial part—Lateral epicondyle of the humerus Deep part---Supinator crest of the ulna	Lateral, anterior, and posterior surfaces of the proximal third of the radius	Deep branch of the radial nerve(C7,C8)	Supinates the forearm and hand
Extensor	Posterior surface of the	Extensor expansion of	Posterior interosseous	Extends the index

indicis	distal third of the ulna and adjacent interosseous membrane	index finger	nerve(C7,**C8**)	finger	
Abductor pollicis longus	Posterior surface of the upper part of the ulna, interosseous membrane, radius(distal to the insetion of the supinator)	Base of the first metacarpal bone	Posterior interosseous nerve(**C7**,C8)	Abducts and extends the thumb at the carpometacarpal joint	
Extensor pollicis brevis	Posterior surface of the radius distal to the abductor pollicis longus and interosseous membrane	Dorsal aspect of the base of the proximal phalanx of thumb	Posterior interosseous nerve(**C7**,C8)	Extends the proximal phalanx of thumb at metacarpophalangeal joint Extends the carpometacarpal joint of the thumb	
Extensor pollicis longus	Posterior surface of the middle third of the ulna and adjacent interosseous membrane	Dorsal aspect of base of the distal phalanx of the thumb	Posterior interosseous nerve(**C7**,C8)	Extends the interphalangeal joint of the thumb,1st metacarpophalangeal joint, and 1st carpometacarpal joint	

N.B. **The deep branch of the radial nerve** passes between the superficial and deep parts of the supinator

The supinator muscle forms the lateral part of the floor of the **cubital**

fossa

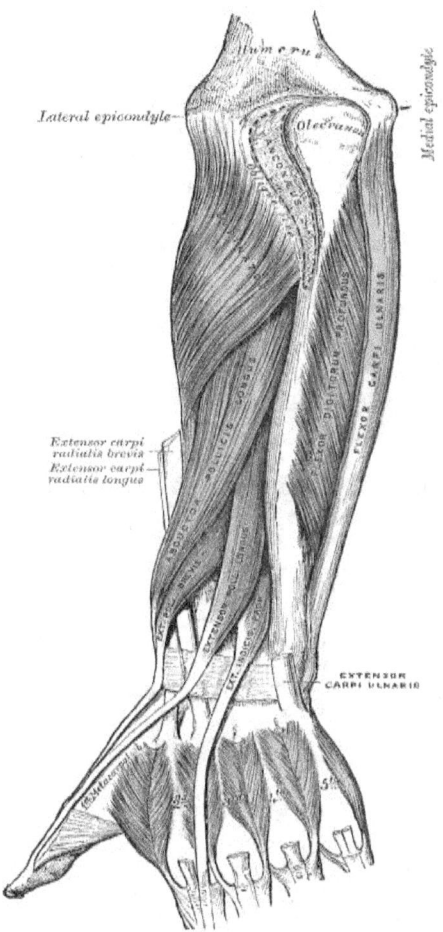

Figure: Deep muscles at the back of the forearm (Wikipedia.org; Free Encyclopedia)

The posterior interosseous nerve is the continuation of the deep branch of the radial nerve at the lower border of the supinator muscle.

Relations of Pronator Teres Muscle

The pronator teres originates from the medial epicondyle of the humerus (superficial head) and the coronoid process of the ulna (deep head). It inserts into the middle of the lateral surface of the shaft of the radius.

1. The median nerve passes between the superficial and deep heads of the pronator teres.

2. The ulnar artery passes deep to the deep head of the pronator teres.

3. The radial artery passes over the lower part of the pronator teres.

Interosseous Membrane

The interosseous membrane is a thin fibrous sheet that connects the adjacent borders (interosseous borders) of the radius and ulna nearly all of their length. The collagen fibers within the interosseous membrane pass mostly inferiorly from lateral to medial direction (radius to ulna).

The interosseous membrane has a free upper margin and a small aperture in its lower end for the passage of the blood vessels.

Functions of the interosseous membrane.

1. The interosseous membrane connects the radius and ulna without hampering pronation and supination.

2. The interosseous membrane provides origin for muscles in the flexor and extensor compartments of the forearm.

3. It provides weight transmission from the radius to ulna and eventually from the hand to the humerus.

Dorsum and Palm of the Hand

The Anatomical Snuff Box

The anatomical snuff box is a triangular depression on the posterolateral side of the wrist and first metacarpal bone.The anatomical snuff box is more distinct when the thumb is extended.

The anatomical snuff box is **bounded on the ulnar side (medially)** by the tendon of extensor pollicis longus. It is bounded laterlly by the tendons of abductor pollicis longus and extensor pollicis brevis. Proximally it is bounded by the distal end of the radial styloid process and distally it is bounded by the proximal part of the first metacarpal bone.

The **floor** of the anatomical snuff box is formed by the scaphoid, trapezium and base of the first metacarpal bone.

The **roof** of the anatomical snuff box is formed by the skin and superficial fascia.

Contents of the anatomical snuff box

1. Terminal parts of the superficial branch of the radial nerve (pass subcutaneously over the snuffbox)

2. The radial artery (passes deep to the extensor tendons of the thumb over the scaphoid and trapezium)

3. Origin of the cephalic vein (from the dorsal venous arch of the hand)

Objective Questions

Q 1. Where is the location of the anatomical snuff box? What are the boundaries of the anatomical snuff box?

Q 2. Which structures form the floor of the anatomical snuff box? What are the contents of the anatomical snuff box?

The Extensor Retinaculum of the Wrist

The extensor retinaculum is an obliquely placed band formed by the thickening of the deep fascia on the back of the wrist. The extensor tendons with their synovial sheaths reach into the hand on the medial, lateral, and posterior surfaces of the wrist in six compartments bounded by the extensor retinaculum.

Attachments:

Laterally, to the lower part of the anterior border of the radius

Medially, to the styloid process of the ulna, the triquetral and the pisiform bones

Tendons in different cubicles under the extensor retinaculum from lateral to medial:

Cubicles	Structures
1.	a. Abductor pollicis longus and b. Extensor pollicis brevis
2.	a. Extensor carpi radialis longus and b. Extensor carpi radialis brevis

3.	Extensor pollicis longus
4.	a. Extensor digitorum b. Extensor indicis c. Posterior interosseous nerve and d. Anterior interosseous nerve
5.	Extensor digiti minimi
6.	Extensor carpi ulnaris

Clinical Notes: De Quervain's tenovaginitis (aka tenosynovitis)

This is a stenosing tenovaginitis that may be due to excessive friction of the tendons in the first cubicle under the extensor retinaculum. The exact cause is not always known. There is palpable thickening of the tendon sheath with pain of the thumb. Treatment is surgical division of the thickened sheath.

Dorsal Wrist Ganglion (synovial cyst)

It is a synovial, nontender, cystic swelling that appears on the dorsum of the wrist or hand. Flexion of the wrist makes the swelling larger, and extension of the wrist tends to make it smaller. Occasionally, the ganglion may develop on the flexor aspect of the wrist, compresses the median nerve and causes carpal tunnel syndrome.

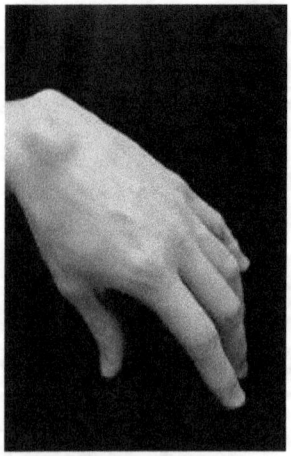

Figure: Ganglion on the dorsum of the hand (Wikipedia.org; Free Encyclopedia)

Rarely, it may be painful. **The ganglion mentioned here is not the collection of nerve cells**. This is the mucoid degeneration of the synovial sheath of the tendons.

Objective Question

What is the structure of a dorsal wrist ganglion?

Dorsal Digital Expansion (extensor expansion or extensor hood)

The **extensor expansion (dorsal expansion, dorsal hood)** is an anatomical term that refers to the flattened tendons of the **extensor digitorum and extensor pollicis longus.** It spans the proximal and distal phalanges.

At the distal end of the metacarpal, the extensor tendon will expand to form a hood, which covers the back and sides of the head of the metacarpal and the proximal phalanx.

The expansion soon divides into three bands:

- The lateral bands pass on either side of the proximal phalanx and stretches all the way to the distal phalanx. The lumbricals of the hand, extensor indicis muscle, dorsal interossei, and palmar interossei insert on these bands.

- A single median band passes down the middle of the finger along the back of the proximal phalanx, ending at the base of the middle phalanx.

- A band known as the retinacular ligament runs obliquely along the middle phalanx, and connects the fibrous digital sheath on the anterior side of the phalanges to the extensor expansion.

Location of the dorsal digital expansion: Dorsal aspect of the proximal phalanges extending from the metacarpophalangeal joint to the distal interphalangeal joints.

Muscles attaching to the dorsal digital expansion of the index, middle, ring and little fingers: the lumbricals, interossei, abductor digiti minimi, extensor indicis and extensor digiti minimi muscles.

Muscles attaching to the dorsal digital expansion of the middle finger: Two dorsal interosseous muscles one from each side, the second lumbrical along the lateral side.

There is no palmer interosseoi attachment to the middle finger. The dorsal interossei are abductors and palmer interossei are adductors. Thus the middle finger cannot be adducted.

Muscles attaching to the dorsal digital expansion of the thumb: adductor pollicis and abductor pollicis brevis

The **action of intrinsic muscles of the hand** (lumbricals, interossei, abductor digiti minimi, adductor pollicis, and abductor pollicis brevis) **through the dorsal digital expansion** is to 1. Flexion of the metacarpophalangeal joint and 2. Extension the interphalangeal joint.

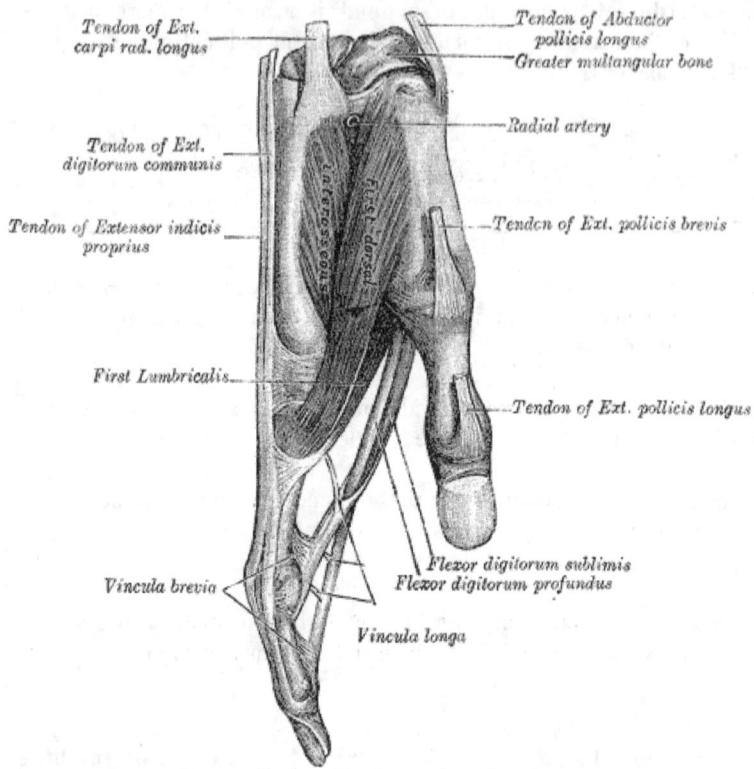

Figure: Mode of insertion tendons on the finger (Wikipedia.org; Free Encyclopedia)

Objective Question

How the dorsal digital expansion is formed? Which muscles are inserted on the dorsal digital expansion?

N.B. The thumb has one interphalangeal joint only

The Recurrent Branch of the Median Nerve

The recurrent branch of the median nerve innervates the 1. flexor pollicis brevis 2. abductor pollicis brevis 3. opponens pollicis

The recurrent branch of the median nerve originates from the median nerve near the distal margin of the flexor retinaculum. It passes proximally between the flexor pollicis brevis and abductor pollicis brevis to end in the opponens pollicis.

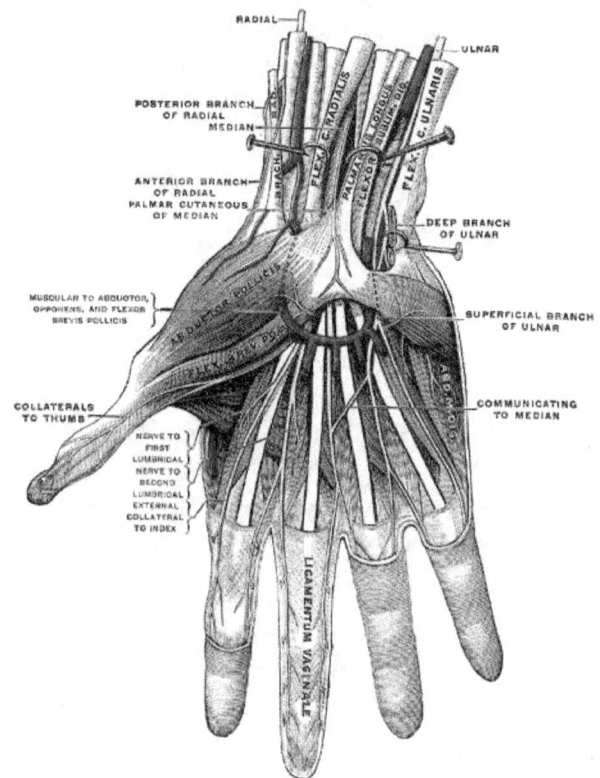

Note: The recurrent branch of the median nerve can be severed in knife wounds where the blades cut across the base of the thenar eminence (Wikipedia.org; Free Encyclopedia)

The Superficial Palmar Arch

The superficial palmar arch is an arterial arch formed primarily by the ulnar artery with contribution from the palmar branch of the radial artery.

Location of the superficial palmar arch: Across the middle of the palm, superficial to the long flexor tendons (tendon of the flexor digitorum longus and flexor digitorum profundus) and deep to the palmar aponeurosis.

Branches of the superficial palmar arch: 1. a palmar digital artery to the medial side of the fifth digit 2. three large common palmar digital arteries for the third, fourth and fifth digits.

Ulnar Nerve in the Hand

The ulnar nerve enters the hand lateral to the pisiform bone and medial to the ulnar artery. Immediately distal to the pisiform bone, it divides into a deep branch, and a superficial branch. All intrinsic muscles of the hand are innervated by deep branch of the ulnar nerve except the three **thenar muscles** (Abductor pollicis brevis, Flexor pollicis brevis, and opponens pollicis) and two lateral lumbricals.The superficial branch of the ulnar nerve innervates the Palmaris brevis. The superficial branch of the ulnar nerve carries cutaneous innervation from the palmar aspect of the medial one and one-half of the digits.

Lesion of the ulnar nerve causes "clawing **of the hands"**, particularly of the medial fingers.

The superficial branch of the ulnar nerve is mainly sensory. It innervates the **Palmaris brevis muscle.**

The deep branch of the ulnar nerve passes deep to the flexor tendons of the hand. It accompanies the deep branch of the ulnar artery.

The deep branch of the ulnar nerve innervates—1. all the **hypothenar muscles** except the palmaris brevis 2. palmar and dorsal interossei 3. adductor pollicis, and 4. Articular branches to the wrist joint.

Guyon's Canal (ulnar canal)

The Guyons's canal is a fibroosseous canal between the hook of the hamate and the pisiform with the medial end of the flexor retinaculum. The deep branch of the ulnar nerve passes through the Guyon's canal.

Rarely, a small out pouching of synovial membrane (ganglion) from the nearby intercarpal joints entraps the ulnar nerve within the Guyon's canal.

Pisiform Bone

The pisiform bone is a sesamoid bone which develops in the tendon of the flexor carpi ulnaris. It articulates with the anterior surface of the triquetrum. The pisiform is not a part of wrist joint.

Allen's Test

The Allen test gives the picture of anastomosis between the radial and ulnar arteries. Both the radial and ulnar arteries are compressed at the wrist. Then pressure is released from one or the other. The pattern of filling of the hand is ascertained. If there is connection between the deep and superficial palmar arteries, only the thumb and radial side of the index finger becomes red, (fill with blood), when force on the radial artery alone is released.

The Flexor Retinaculum (Transverse Carpal Ligament)

The flexor retinaculum is a tough fibrous band which crosses the front of the carpal arch and converts its concavity into the carpal tunnel. This ligament **connects the pisiform and hook of the hamate medially by the tubercles of the scaphoid and trapezium laterally**.

The flexor retinaculum **holds** the flexor tendons at the wrist and **prevents** them from bowing.

The tendons of the **Palmaris longus and flexor carpi ulnaris** partially inserts into the anterior surface of the retinaculum. Distally some of the **intrinsic muscles** of the thumb and little finger originate from the retinaculum.

The flexor retinaculum lies deep to the ulnar nerve and the ulnar artery and superficial to the median nerve.

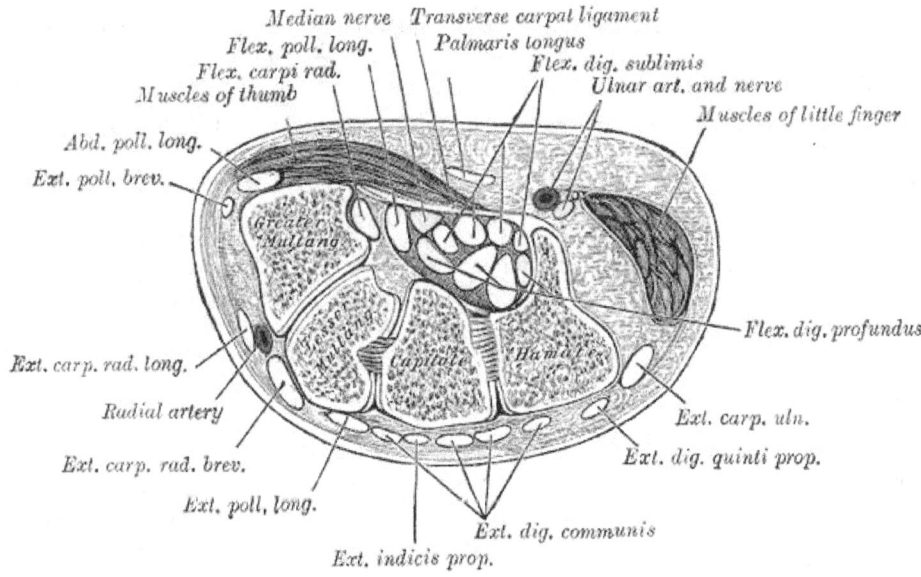

Figure: The carpal tunnel and its contents (Wikipedia.org; Free Encyclopedia)

Carpal Tunnel Syndrome

The carpal tunnel is a passageway on the anterior side of the wrist. Carpal tunnel syndrome is caused by a compression of the median nerve within the carpal tunnel. It is made of the carpal bones which are covered by the flexor retinaculum. It contains the tendons of flexor pollicis longus, flexor digitorum superficialis, flexor digitorum profundus, and the median nerve. All the tendons of the flexor digitorum profundus and flexor digitorum superficialis are surrounded by a single synovial sheath. The tendon of the flexor pollicis longus is surrounded by a separate synovial sheath. The median nerve is anterior to the tendons in the carpal tunnel. If the sheath over the common flexor tendons, the ulnar bursa, becomes inflamed, this could compress the median nerve in the tunnel, leading to pain and weakness in the hand. Weakness and loss of muscle mass of the thenar muscles may also occur.

The **cause of carpal tunnel syndrome** is often unclear. It may be caused by a number of things. For instance, overuse, rheumatoid arthritis, pregnancy, cysts arising from the carpal joints, and hypothyroidism.

Treatment: Rest, reduction of inflammation and edema in the carpal tunnel. Surgical resection of the flexor retinaculum may be required.

Symptoms of carpal tunnel syndrome

The symptoms usually start slowly, with frequent burning, tingling, or numbness in the palm of the hand and the fingers, especially the thumb and the index and middle fingers. The symptoms often first come out in one or both hands during the night, since many people sleep with flexed wrists. As symptoms worsen, people might feel tingling during the day. Decreased grip strength may make it hard to form a fist, grasp small objects, or perform other manual tasks. Patient usually complaints pain along the distribution of the median nerve. The thenar muscles may be wasted (**Ape hand**). The patient has inability to oppose the thumb.

 There is an **absence of tactile sensation** may exist on the lateral two-thirds of the palm, palmer surfaces of the thumb, index, middle, ring (lateral half) fingers. Some people are unable to tell the difference between hot and cold stimulation by touch.

.

Tinel's Sign:

Gently tapping over the flexor retinaculum produces symptoms of carpal tunnel syndrome (**Positive sign** is pain and tingling along the distribution of the median nerve in the hand)

Phalen's sign:

The Phalen or wrist-flexion test involves having the patient hold his or her forearms upright by pointing the fingers down and pressing the backs of the hands together. The presence of carpal tunnel syndrome is suggested if one or more symptoms, such as tingling or increasing numbness are felt in the fingers within 1 minute.

MCQ

Q.Which muscles most typically become weakened in carpal tunnel syndrome?

A. Palmer interossei

B. Dorsal interossei

C. **Thenar**

D. Hypothenar

E. Third and fourth lumbricals

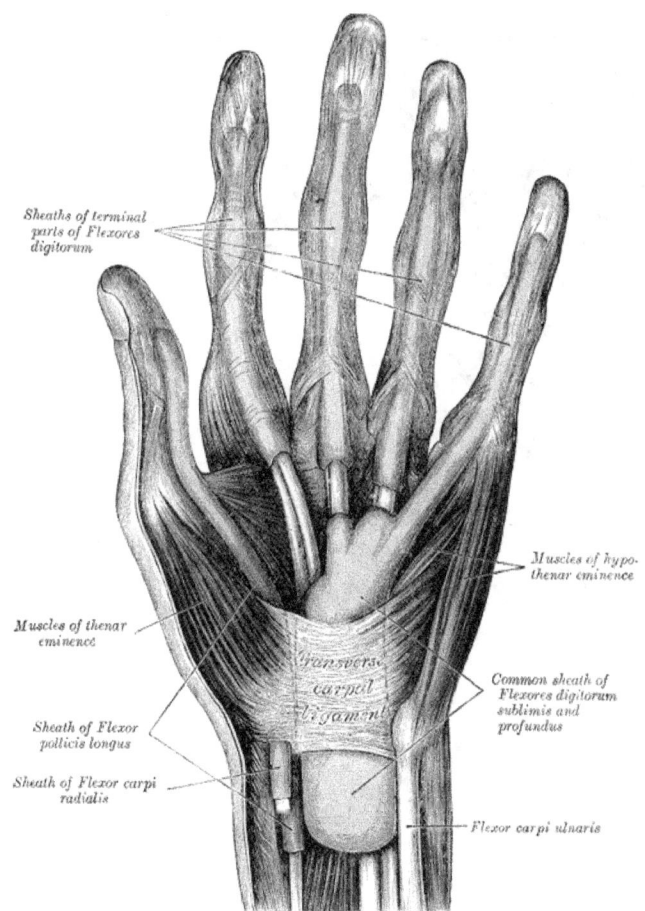

Figure: Tendons and synovial sheath of the hand (Wikipedia.org; Free Encyclopedia)

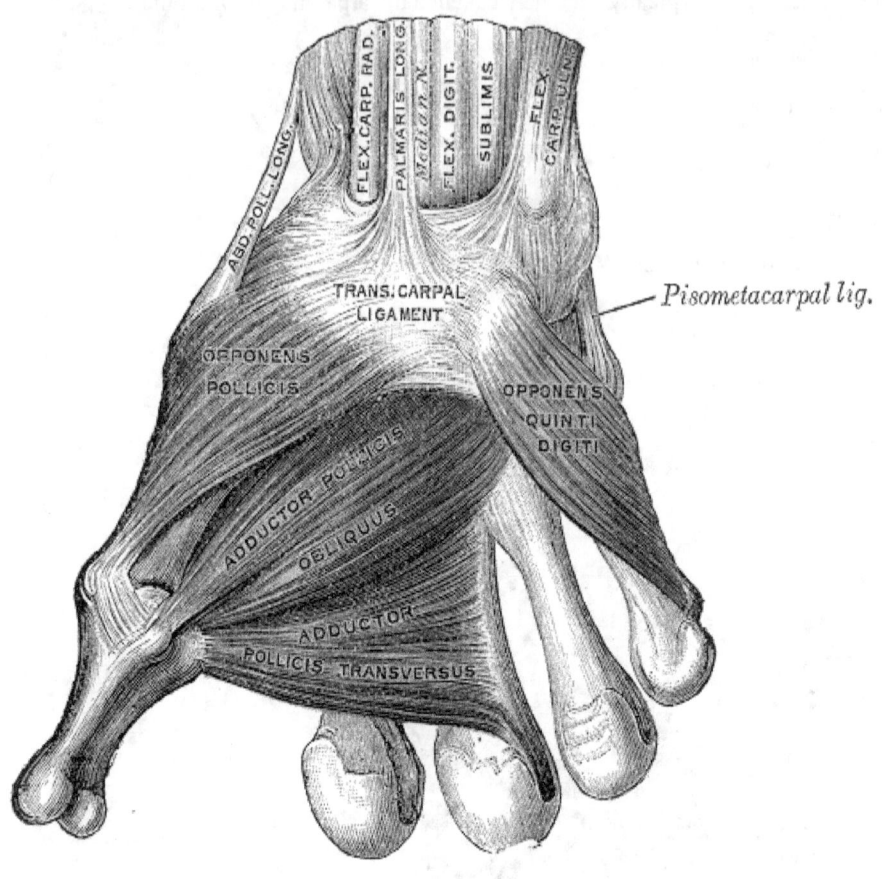

Figure: Muscles and tendons of the hand (Wikipedia.org; Free Encyclopedia)

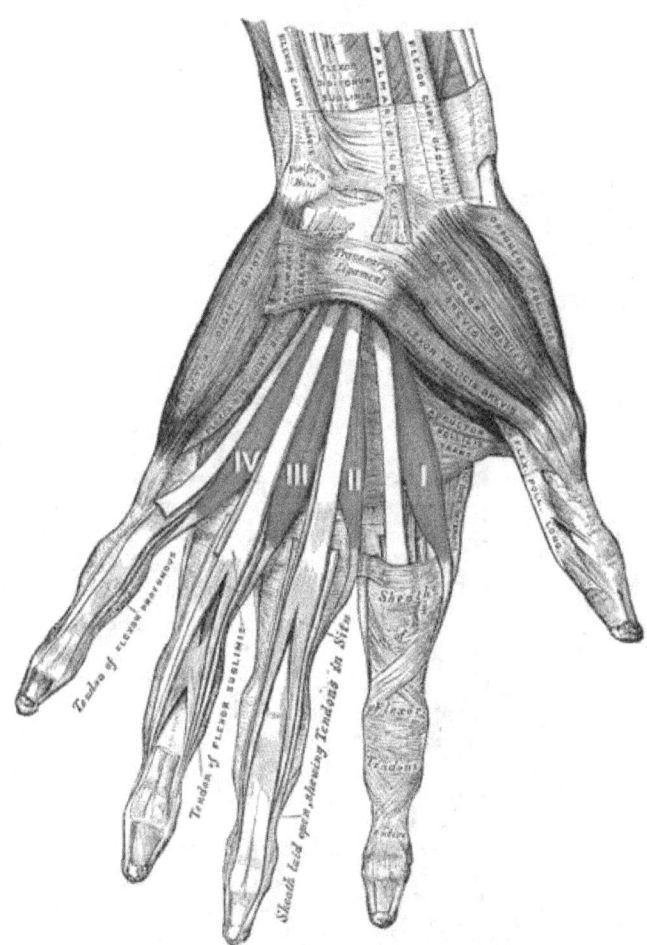

Figure: Muscles and tendons of the palm (Wikipedia.org; Free Encyclopedia)

Objective Questions

Q 1.What is the attachment of the flexor retinaculum? What is its function? What structures passes beneath the flexor retinaculum?

Q 2. What is carpal tunnel syndrome? What are the motor and sensory symptoms seen in carpal tunnel syndrome?

Course of Radial Artery in the Wrist and Hand

The radial artery passes laterally beneath the brachioradialis tendon with the superficial radial nerve. This artery passes over the anatomical snuff-box and reaches the palm by entering between the two heads of the first dorsal interosseous muscle. The artery then divides into the princeps pollicis artery and the deep palmar arch.

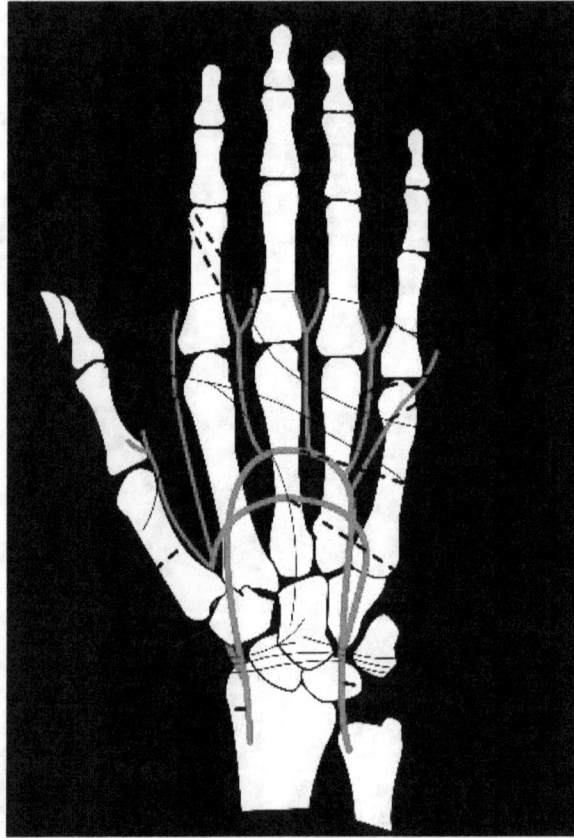

1. Princeps pollicis

This branch of the radial artery passes under the flexor pollicis longus and divides into two proper digital arteries to the thumb

2. Radialis indicis. This branch of the radial artery passes along the lateral side of the index finger.

3. **Deep palmar arch.** The deep palmar arch lies upon the bases of the metacarpal bones and on the interossei of the hand, being covered by the oblique head of the adductor pollicis muscle, the flexor tendons of the fingers, and the lumbricals of the hand. It is usually formed mainly from the terminal part of the radial artery, with the ulnar artery contributing via its deep palmar branch.

4. Superficial palmar branch. This branch of the radial artery forms the superficial palmar arch with the ulnar artery.

Figure: 1.The deep palmar arch (located proximally) and 2. The superficial palmar arch (located distally) (Wikipedia.org; Free Encyclopedia)

Note: Disruption of the radial artery could lead to loss of blood supply to the thumb and lateral half of the index finger if anastomosis with the ulnar artery is not adequate to maintain supply.

Ulnar Artery Branches in the Wrist and Hand

Superficial Palmar Arch

The superficial palmar arch is formed by termination of the **ulnar artery** along with the superficial branch of the radial artery. Three common digital arteries come out of the superficial palmar arch. Each of the common digital arteries gives rise to two proper digital arteries. The superficial palmar arch is **more distally located** than the deep palmar arch. If one is to fully extend the thumb and draw a line from the distal border of the thumb across the palm, this would be of the level of the superficial palmar arch. The deep palmar arch is about a finger width proximal to this.

Notes: The Allen's test is used to evaluate adequate anatomoses between the radial and ulnar arteries.

Palmar branch of the median nerve and palmar branch of ulnar nerve passes superficial to the flexor retinaculum.

Palmar branch of median nerve originates from the median nerve in the distal forearm immediately proximal to the flexor retinaculum, passes superficially into the hand and innervates skin over the base and central palm.

The palmar branch of the median nerve is **spared in carpal tunnel syndrome** because it passes superficial to the flexor retinaculum. If the function of the palmer branch of the median nerve is compromised in the carpal tunnel, then the lesion of the median nerve is proximal to the wrist.

The palmar branch of the ulnar nerve originates in the middle of the forearm and passes into the hand to supply the skin on the medial side of the palm.

The Median Nerve in the Hand

The median nerve **enters the hand by passing through the carpal tunnel** and splits into a recurrent branch and four palmar digital branches.

The median nerve is responsible for the **opposition of the thumb** to the other digits.

The palmar branch of the median nerve from forearm carries cutaneous sensation from the palm. The palmar digital branches of the median nerve carry cutaneous sensation from the palmar surface of the lateral two thirds of the palm, palmar surface of the thumb, index finger, lateral half of ring finger, and dorsal aspect of the distal phalanges (nailbeds) of the same digits.

In addition, the digital branches of the median nerve supply the two lateral lumbrical muscles.

The recurrent branch of the median nerve innervates three thenar muscles---1. Abductor pollicis brevis 2. Flexor pollicis brevis and 3. Opponens pollicis brevis

The recurrent branch of the median nerve begins from the median nerve near the distal margin of the flexor retinaculum. It passes proximally over the flexor pollicis brevis, between the flexor pollicis brevis and abductor pollicis brevis to end in opponens pollicis brevis.

Note: The recurrent branch of the median nerve can be cut if a sharp object passes over the base of the thenar eminence.

The **Adductor pollicis**, the only thenar muscle is innervated by the deep branch of the ulnar nerve.

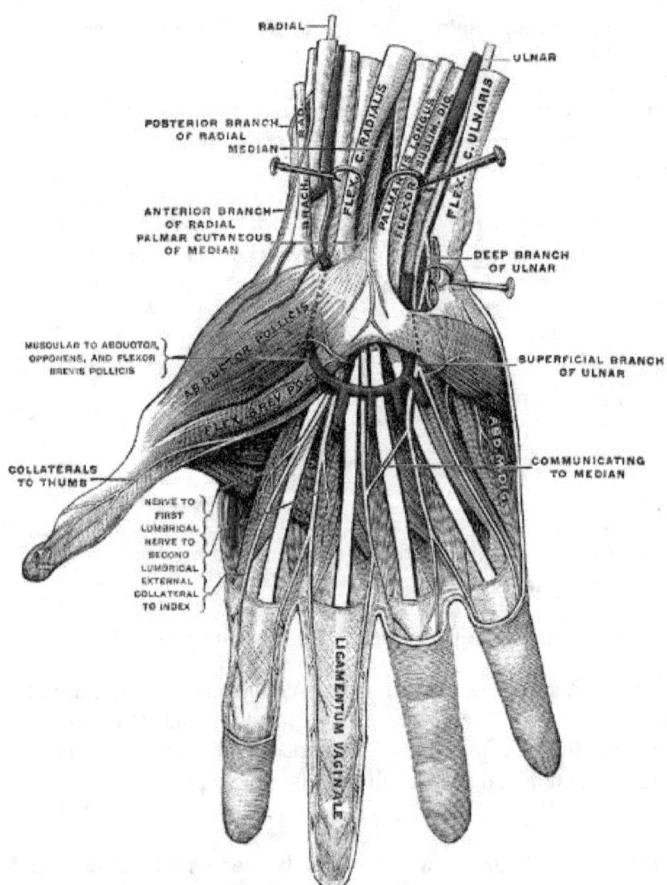

(Wikipedia.org; Free Encyclopedia)

Functions of the Lumbricals of Hand

The lumbricals flex the metacarpophalangeal joints and extend the interphalangeal joints of the index, ring, middle, and little fingers. Dysfunction of the lumbrical muscles contributes to "**clawing** of the hand".

The Superficial Branch of the Ulnar Nerve

The superficial branch of the ulnar nerve innervates the palmar brevis muscle and continues across the palm to innervate the skin of the ulnar side of the palm.

Palmar Aponeurosis

The palmar aponeurosis is the thickening of the deep fascia on the palm. It is triangular in shape. The apex of the palmar aponeurosis is attached to the tendon of the Palmaris longus and the flexor retinaculum. The base of the palmar aponeurosis is blended to the skin at the base of the digits. **Tendons, nerves, and blood vessels of the palm lie deep to the palmar aponeurosis**.

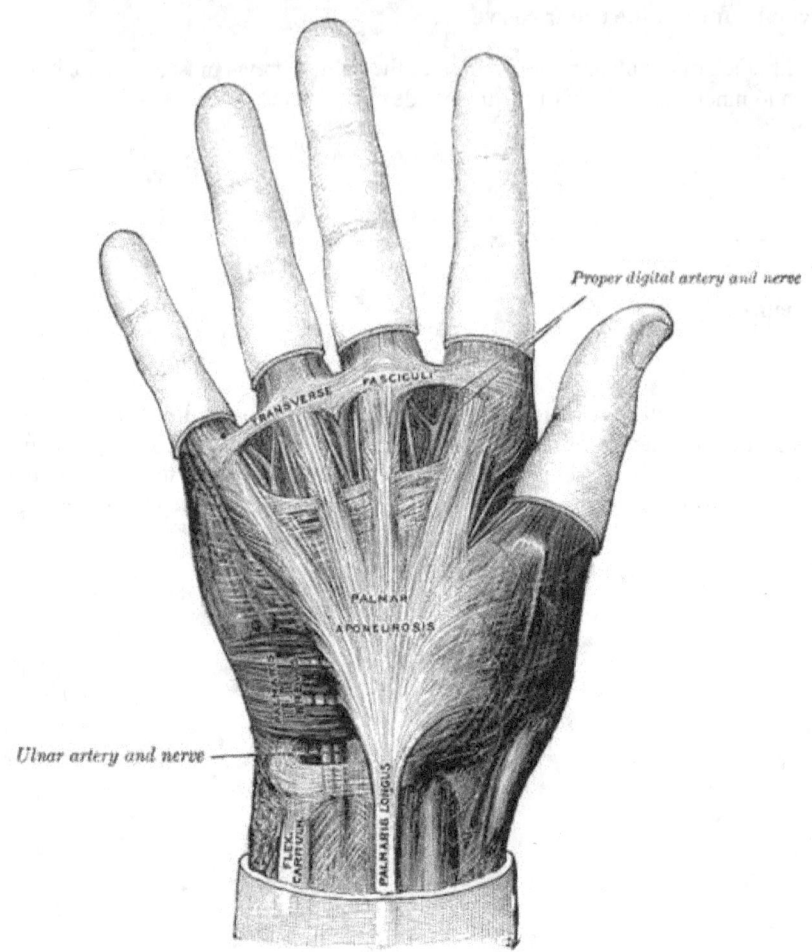

(Wikipedia.org; Free Encyclopedia)

Functions of the Palmar Aponeurosis:

1. The palmar aponeurosis protects the underlying structures.

2. The palmar aponeurosis gives attachment to the muscles (e.g. Palmaris longus and Palmaris brevis)

3. It improves the grip of the hand by firmly attaching the skin.

Dupuytren's Contracture (Dupuytren's Disease).

This is the fibrous contracture and nodule formation in the medial aspect of the palmar fascia and palmar aponeurosis. The ring finger and the little fingers are affected with flexion deformities of the metacarpophalangeal and proximal interphalangeal joints. The Dupuytren's Contracture is seen in elderly person. The exact cause is not known. The typical patient is a white male over the age of 40. Smoking and diabetes mellitus are contributing factors. This is highly correlated with coronary artery disease, perhaps due to vasospasm caused by sympathetic innervations of the vasculature within the T1 component of the ulnar nerve. **Management** is surgical.

Palmaris Longus Tendon

The palmaris longus tendon is long and cord like. The Palmaris longus muscle is **absent in about 15% of population**. The Palmaris longus muscle lies between the flexor carpi radialis and flexor carpi ulnaris. The Palmaris longus tendon passes superficial to the flexor retinaculum and attaches to it and to the palmar aponeurosis. At the wrist, the median nerve passes deep and lateral to the Palmaris longus tendon.

To test the Palmaris longus tendon—the tendon is made visible by flexing the wrist joint and touching the pad of little finger by the thumb.

Objective Questions

Q1. Which muscle tendon attaches and crosses the flexor retinaculum?

Q2. How the deep palmar arch is is formed? What is the location of the deep palmar arch? Which muscles tendons pass over the deep palmar arch? Which muscles pass beneath the deep palmar arch?

Q3. Which muscles of the hand are innervated by the recurrent branch of the median nerve?

Flexor Carpi Radialis Tendon

The flexor carpi radialis tendon inserts into the palmar surface of the bases of the second and third metacarpal bones.

In the lower part of the forearm, the radial artery passes between the tendons of the brachioradialis and the flexor carpi radialis.

The flexor carpi radialis tendon passes through a compartment formed by trapezium and a deep slip from the lateral part of the flexor retinaculum.

Intrinsic Muscles of the Hand and their Nerve Supply

Thenar muscles

Name of the muscle	Origin	Insertion	Nerve Supply	Action
Abductor pollicis brevis	Tubercle of the scaphoid and trapezium and flexor retinaculum	Proximal phalanx and extensor hood of the thumb	Recurrent branch of the median nerve(C8 **T1**)	Abducts the thumb at metacarpophalangeal joint
Opponens pollicis	Tubercle of the trapezium and flexor retinaculum	Lateral margin of the first metacarpal bone	Recurrent branch of the median nerve(C8 **T1**)	Medially rotates the thumb
Flexor pollicis brevis	Tubercle of the trapezium and flexor retinaculum	Proximal phalanx of the thumb	Recurrent branch of the median nerve(C8 **T1**)	Flexes the thumb at the metacarpophalangeal joint

Hypothenar muscles

Name of the muscle	Origin	Insertion	Nerve Supply	Action
Opponens digiti minimi	Hook of the hamate and flexor retinaculum	Medial aspect of the 5th metacarpal bone	Deep branch of the ulnar nerve(C8,**T1**)	Draws the little finger into opposition with thumb
Flexor digiti minimi	Hook of the hamate and flexor	Medial side of the base of the proximal	Deep branch of the ulnar nerve(C8,**T1**)	Flexes the 5th metacarpophalangeal joint

brevis	retinaculum	phalanx of little finger		
Abductor digiti minimi	Pisiform and the pisohamate ligament	Medial side of the proximal phalanx of the little finger	Deep branch of the ulnar nerve(C8,**T1**)	Abduct the little finger at metacarpophalangeal joint

Other intrinsic muscles of the hand

Name of the muscle	Origin	Insertion	Nerve Supply	Action
Adductor pollicis	Transverse head—anterior surface of the shaft of the 3rd metacarpal bone Oblique head—capitates, bases of the 2nd and 3rd metacarpal bones	Medial side of base of proximal phalanx of thumb	Deep branch of the ulnar nerve(C8 ,**T1**)	Adducts the thumb
Palmar brevis	Medial side of palmar aponeurosis and flexor retinaculum	Skin of medial side of palm	Superficial branch of the ulnar nerve	Improves grip Makes wrinkles on the medial aspect of palm
Palmar interossei (4 unipennate muscles)	Sides of the 1st,2nd, 4th, and 5th metacarpal bones	Proximal phalanx of the 1st,2nd,4th, and 5th fingers and into the respective dorsal digital expansion	Deep branch of the ulnar nerve(C8 ,**T1**)	Adducts the fingers, flexes the metacarpophalangeal joints, and extends interphalangeal joints
Dorsal interossei(4 bipennate muscles)	Sides of the metacarpal bones	Proximal phalanx of the index, middle and ring fingers	Deep branch of the ulnar nerve(C8 ,**T1**)	Abducts the index, middle and ring fingers, flexes the metacarpophalangeal joints,

		and into the respective dorsal digital expansion		and extends the interphalangeal joints of the index, middle and ring fingers
Lumbricals (lumbrical means worm-like)	Tendons of flexor digitorum profundus	Lateral sides of the dorsal digital expansions	1st and 2nd lumbricals by the median nerve 3rd and 4th lumbricals by the ulnar nerve	Flexes the metacarpophal angeal joint and extends the interphalangeal joints

Notes: The dorsal interossei abduct the 2nd to 4th digits. The palmer interossei adducts 2nd, 4th, and 5th digits relative to the 3rd digit. All the interossei muscles are innervated by the ulnar nerve.

The lumbricals connects the flexor tendons with extensor tendons. The first and second lumbricals are **unipennate**. The third and fourth lumbricals are **bipennate.**

The ability to adduct the digits against resistance is used to **test the motor function of the deep branch of the ulnar nerve**.

The adductor **pollicis muscle** is a muscle in the hand that functions to adduct the thumb. It has two heads: transverse and oblique. **The radial artery** passes between the two heads, travelling from the back of the hand into the palm, where it forms the **deep palmar arch**. Between the oblique and transverse heads is a thin fibrous arcade which the deep branch of the ulnar nerve passes as it traverses the palm laterally.The deep branch of the ulnar nerve is accompanied by the deep palmar arch. **Froment's sign** is a special test of the wrist. It tests for palsy of the ulnar nerve, specifically; the action of adductor pollicis. **Froment's sign** is used to test for a compromised adductor pollicis muscle.

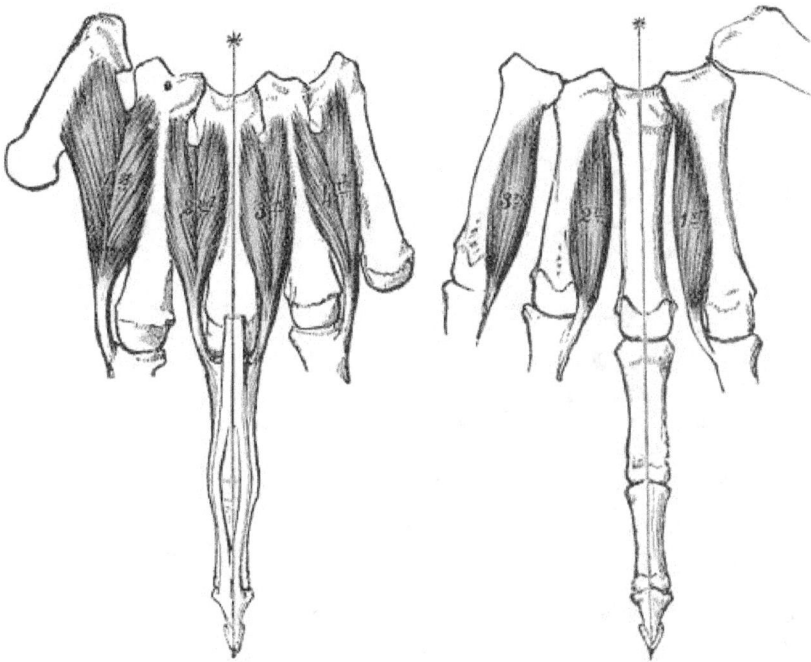

(Wikipedia.org; Free Encyclopedia)

MCQs

Q1. Thickening and contracture of which of the following causes Dupuytren's Contracture?

A. Antebrachial fascia

B. Brachial fascia

C. **Palmar fascia and palmar aponeurosis**

D. Clavipectoral fascia

Q2. Which of the following muscles of the hand connects the flexor tendon with extensor tendons?

A. Palmaris brevis

B. Adductor brevis

C. Dorsal interossei

D. Palmar interossei

E. Lumbricals

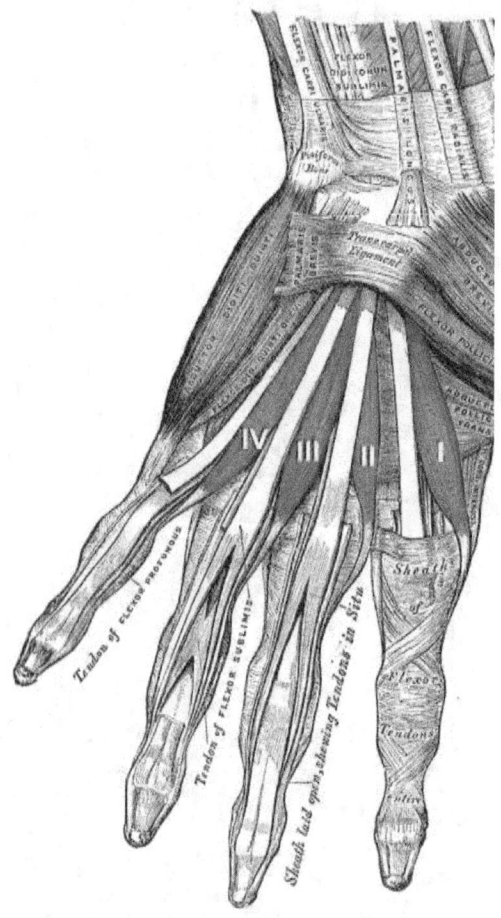

Figure: Small muscles of the hand. The limbricals are leveled as I, II, III, and IV from lateral to medial(Wikipedia.org; Free Encyclopedia)

Notes:

The lumbricals take origin from the tendon of the flexor digitorum profundus.

The lumbrical muscles connect the flexor digitorum profundus tendon to the extensor hood.

The two lateral lumbricals are unipinnate muscles.

The two medial lumbricals are bipennate muscles.

The axial line for adduction and abduction passes through the middle finger

The middle finger has abduction movement only because the axial line passes through it.

3PAD—Three palmar interossei cause **ADDUCTION**

4DAB---Four dorsal interossei cause **ABDUCTION**

The lumbricals flexes the metacarcophalangeal joints and extends the interphalangeal joints of the index, middle, ring, and little fingers.

The interossei muscles assist in the action of lumbrical by flexing the metacarpophalangeal joint and extending the interphalangeal joints.

The lumbricals are used during writing.

The two medial lumbricals are innervated by the deep branch of the ulnar nerve.

The two lateral lumbricals are innervated by the palmar digital branches of the median nerve.

The cutaneous innervation of the anatomical snuff box is carried by the superficial branch of the radial nerve.

The palmaris brevis is innervated by the superficial branch of the ulnar nerve.

The palmar interossei has no attachment to the middle finger and third metacarpal bone.

The dorsal interossei has bilateral attachment to the middle finger.

The thumb has two phalanges only.

Differences between the Palmar and Dorsal interossei Muscles

	Palmer interossei	**Dorsal interossei**
Location	**On the palmer surface of the metacarpal bones**	**Between the metacarpal bones**
Size	**Smaller**	**Larger**
Number of head for each muscle	**One (unipennate muscle)**	**Two (bipennate muscle)**

Function	Adducts the fingers	Abducts the fingers
Attachment to 3rd metacarpal and middle finger	Absent	Present

Differences between 1st and 2nd (radial) from the 3rd and 4th (ulnar) lumbricals

	1st and 2nd Lumbricals	3rd and 4th Lumbricals
Location	Radial side	Ulnar side
Insertion	Base of the distal phalanx of the middle and index finger	Base of the distal phalanx of the little and ring finger
Innervation	Ulnar nerve	Median nerve

Note: Loss of function of the lumbrical muscles gives rise to "clawing" of the hand.

Boxer's fracture

Boxers's fractures are associated with punching injuries.Typically there is an oblique fracture through the neck of the fifth metacarpal bone.The knuckle of the little finger is lost. Other metacarpals may also be fractured. This is also called brawler's **fracture or bar room fracture**.

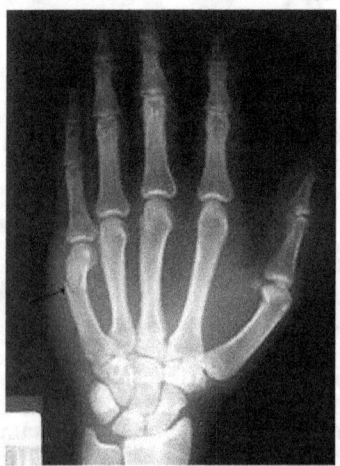

Figure: The black arrow indicates the fracture line in boxer's fracture (Wikipedia.org; Free Encyclopedia)

In sports medicine, **mallet finger**, also **baseball finger, dropped finger** and (more generally) **extensor tendon injury**, is an injury of the extensor digitorum tendon of the fingers at the distal interphalangeal joint (DIP). It results when a ball (such as a softball, basketball, or volleyball) is miscaught or a finger is jammed into the base pad. The extensor mechanism is disrupted. The finger is held flexed at the distal interphalangeal joint. There is no active movement but passive movement is unimpaired. In time, the proximal phalanx may become hyperextended.

Treatment options include putting the finger in a Mallet **splint** for 6 to 8 weeks.This allows the extensor tendon to reattach to the base of the distal interphalangeal joint. If the finger is bent during these weeks the healing process must start all over again.

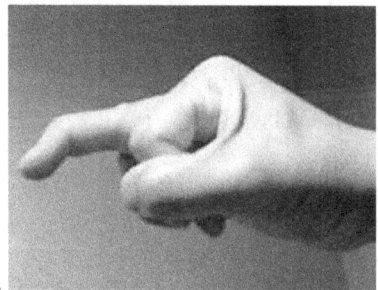

Figure: Mallet finger is indicated in the middle finger in this photograph. Note how the tip of the finger bends downwards while the rest of the finger stays straight. (Wikipedia.org; Free Encyclopedia)

Objective Questions

Q 1. What is the nerve supply of the adductor pollicis?

Q 2. The thenar muscles are innervated by nerves derived from which cord of the brachial plexus?

Q 3. What are the actions of the a. lumbricals b. dorsal interossei and c. palmar interossei? What are the differences between the palmer and dorsal interossei muscles?

Q 4. From which tendons the lumbricals arise? What are the differences between the lateral and medial lumbricals?

Q 5. Which muscles of the hand are innervated by the median nerve?

Mode of insertion of Flexor Digitorum Superficialis and Flexor Digitorum Profundus.

Near the base of the proximal phalanx of each finger, the tendon of the flexor digitorum superficialis splits and reunites around each side of the tendon of flexor digitorum profundus and eventually inserts to the sides of the middle phalanx.

On the flexor surface of the proximal phalanges of the index, middle, ring, and little finger, the flexor digitorum profundus passes through an opening formed in the covering tendon of the flexor digitorum superficialis muscle and passes distally to insert into the anterior surface of the base of the distal phalanx.

Vincula

These are **synovial folds** which attach to the superficial and deep flexors of the middle and distal phalanges and provide blood supply to these tendons. Inflammation associated with tenosynovitis may constrict the blood supply, causing ischemic necrosis of the tendons.

There are two types of vincula---1. vincula longa and 2. vincula brevis

The Common Synovial Sheath (common flexor tendon sheath)

The common synovial sheath for the flexor digitorum superficialis and flexor digitorum profundus is called the **ulnar bursa**. The synovial sheath for the flexor pollicis longus is called the **radial bursa**. These bursae extend from the distal end of the flexor aspect of the forearm to the middle of the palm. The tendons for the index, middle, and ring finger fan out and enter their respective **digital synovial sheath**. The common synovial sheath is continuous with the digital synovial sheath of little finger and occasionally with the digital synovial sheath of the thumb.

Clinical note: **Finger prick** to get blood for diagnostic purposes should be done on the ring, middle, or index fingers only. Finger prick on the thumb and little finger may spread the infection proximal to the flexor retinaculum and can cause **carpal tunnel syndrome**. The infection may spread to the space of **Parona** (the space between the pronator quadrates and the overlying flexor tendons).

Objective Questions

Q. Define a. radial bursa b. ulnar bursa and c. space of Parona

MCQ

Q. A 30-year-old farmer cut his thumb while harvesting. The wound was contaminated with soil. A few days later he developed pain and swelling along entire thumb extending to the wrist. Which of following synovial sheath of tendon is most likely inflamed?

A. Flexor digitorum superficialis

B. Flexor digitorum profundus

C. Flexor carpi ulnaris

D. Flexor Pollicis longus

Compartment Syndrome and Volkmann's Ischemic Contracture

Deep fascia of the forearm has limited elasticity. Any buildup of fluid under the deep fascia due to trauma (supracondylar fracture) or burn can lead to increased tension and pain in the compartment. If the pressure is high enough, tissue perfusion pressure will be compromised. This will lead to **compartment syndrome**. There will be ischemia and necrosis of the muscles.Supracondylar fracture also causes spasm of the bracial artery and thereby causes further ischemia. Damage to the muscles is irreversible. Muscle fibers become atrophic, contracted, and replaced by fibrous tissue (**Volkmann's ischemic contracture**)

Common sites of Compartment Syndrome—1. Anterior compartment of the forearm 2. The intrinsic muscles of hand 3. The lower leg.

Management:
 Surgical decompression.

Median Artery

The median artery is a branch of the anterior interosseous artery. The median artery accompanies and supplies the median nerve as far as the palm.

Deep Branch of the Radial Nerve and Posterior Interosseous Nerve

The radial nerve divides into deep and superficial branches at the level of the lateral epicondyle of the humerus.

The deep branch of the radial nerve is entirely muscular and articular in distribution.

The superficial branch of the radial nerve is entirely cutaneous in distribution along the dorsum of the hand and fingers.

The deep branch of the radial nerve innervates the supinator muscle and passes to the posterior compartment of the forearm by passing between the superficial and deep part of the supinator muscle. The deep branch of the radial nerve then continues as the posterior interosseous verve.

N.B. According to Gray's Anatomy, the deep branch of the radial nerve is the same as the posterior interosseous nerve.

Superficial Branch of the Radial Nerve

This is the only part of the radial nerve that enters the hand. The terminal branches of the superficial branch of the radial nerve can be palpated or rolled against the extensor pollicis longus tendon in the anatomical snuff box.

The superficial branch of the radial nerve innervates the skin over the dorsolateral palm and dorsal surface of the lateral three and a half fingers except the terminal phalanx.

Lateral Cutaneous Nerve of the Forearm (lateral antebrachial cutaneous nerve)

The lateral cutaneous nerve of the forearm begins lateral to the tendon of the biceps brachii at the cubital fossa as a continuation of the musculocutaneous nerve. It passes along the lateral aspect of the forearm to the wrist.

Medial Cutaneous Nerve of the Forearm (medial antebrachial cutaneous nerve)

The medial cutaneous nerve of the forearm is an independent branch of the medial cord of the brachial plexus (C8, T1). In the arm the medial cutaneous nerve of the forearm first accompanies the ulnar nerve and then the basilic vein. It divides into anterior and posterior branches before entering the forearm. It carries sensation from the anteromedial aspect of the forearm as far as the wrist.

Notes: There is no anterior cutaneous nerve for the arm and forearm.

The brachial plexus has no anterior cord.

Wartenberg's disease—This is a sensory neuropathy due to entrapment of the superficial branch of the radial nerve beneath the tendon of the brachioradialis. Wartenberg's disease may be a complication of a fracture of the lower part of the radius. This condition is associated with paresthesia or pain of the lateral side of the dorsum of the hand.

Martin—Gruber connection—In approximately 17% of cases motor fibers from median or anterior interosseous nerve communicate with the ulnar nerve and innervate some intrinsic muscles of the hand. Hence distal lesion of the median nerve may not affect the thenar muscles and distal lesion of the ulnar nerve may not affect the hypothenar muscles.

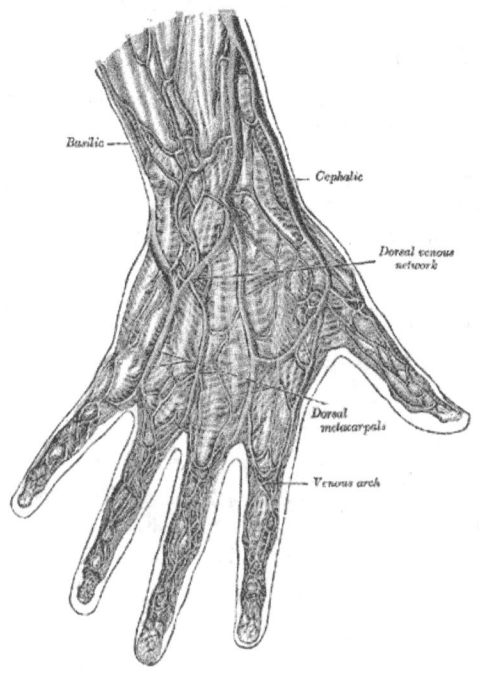

Figure: Formation of the cephalic and basilic vein from the dorsal venous network of the hand (Wikipedia.org; Free Encyclopedia).

The **dorsal venous network** is visible and is accessed for multiple procedures.The dorsal venous networks are **dissimilar** even in the same individual.

Nerves of the Upper Limb

Nerve	Origin	Course	Innervation	Clinical notes
Suprascapular nerve(C5,C6)	**Upper trunk of the brachial plexus**	Runs laterally deep to the trapezius and omohyoid and enters the supraspinos fossa through the suprascapular notch **inferior to the superior transverse scapular**	**Suprascapinatus** muscle **Infraspinatus** muscle **Articular branch to** the shoulder joint and acromioclavicular joint **Rarely** cutaneous	Lesion of the suprascapular nerve is caused by the neuralgic amyotrophy,entrapment neuropathy in the scapular notch or trauma to the shoulder and scapula **There is pain of the shoulder and wasting and weakness of the supraspinatus and**

		ligament. It runs deep to the supraspinatus and curves around the lateral border of the spine of the scapula with suprascapular artery and **reaches the infraspinous fossa.**	branch to proximal arm	**infraspinatus.** **There is inability to initiate abduction of the arm at the shoulder joint and to decreased ability to rotate the arm externally.**
Nerve to subclavius(C4, C5, and **C6**)	Upper trunk of the brachial plexus near the junction of the 5th and 6th cervical ventral rami	It descends **anteriorly** over the brachial plexus , subclavian vessels,and pierces the subclavius muscle	Subclavius	It is usually connected to the phrenic nerve
Long thoracic nerve(C5-C7)	Roots of the brachial plexus	It passes **behind** the brachial plexus and descends along the lateral border of the serratus anterior	Serratus anterior	**Winging of the scapula** is the manifestation of the long thoracic nerve lesion
Intercostobrachial nerve	**Second** or third intercostal nerve(**lateral cutaneous branch**)	**Pierces** the intercostals and serratus anterior muscle at the midaxillary line and may communicate with the medial brachial	**Sensory innervations** to the upper part of the posteromedial aspect of the arm and axillary skin	Associated with **cardiac referred** pain. Contains **postganglionic** sympathetic fibers

		cutaneous nerve		
Supraclavicular nerve		Passes anterior to the clavicle, immediately deep to the platysma	Supply the skin over the clavicle and superolateral aspect of the pectoralis major.	
Superficial branch of the radial nerve		It enters the hand by crossing over the anatomical snuff box on the dorsolateral aspect of the wrist	Skin over the lateral aspect of the palm close the anatomical snuff box, lateral 2/3rd of the dorsum of the hand, and lateral three and one half digits distally to approximately the terminal interphalangeal joints	The only part of the radial nerve that goes into the hand is the superficial branch. The superficial branch of the radial nerve can be palpated or rolled against the tendon of the extensor pollicis longus in the anatomical snuff box.

Cutaneous innervations of the upper limb

The cutaneous innervations of the upper limb include the following:

1. The supraclavicular nerves (C3, C4)

2. The upper lateral cutaneous nerve of the arm (C5, C6)

3. The lower lateral cutaneous nerve of the arm (C5, C6)

4. The intercostobrachial nerve (T2)

5. The medial cutaneous nerve of the arm (T1, T2)

6. The posterior cutaneous nerve of the arm (C5)

7. The lateral antebrachial cutaneous nerve of the forearm {the lateral cutaneous nerve of the forearm} (C5, C6)

8. The medial antebrachial cutaneous nerve {the medial cutaneous nerve of the forearm} (C8, T1)

9. The posterior cutaneous nerve of the forearm (C6-C8)

10. Cutaneous branches of the median nerve (C6-C8)

11. Cutaneous branches of the ulnar nerve (C7-C8)

12. Cutaneous branches from the superficial terminal branches of the radial nerve (C6-C8)

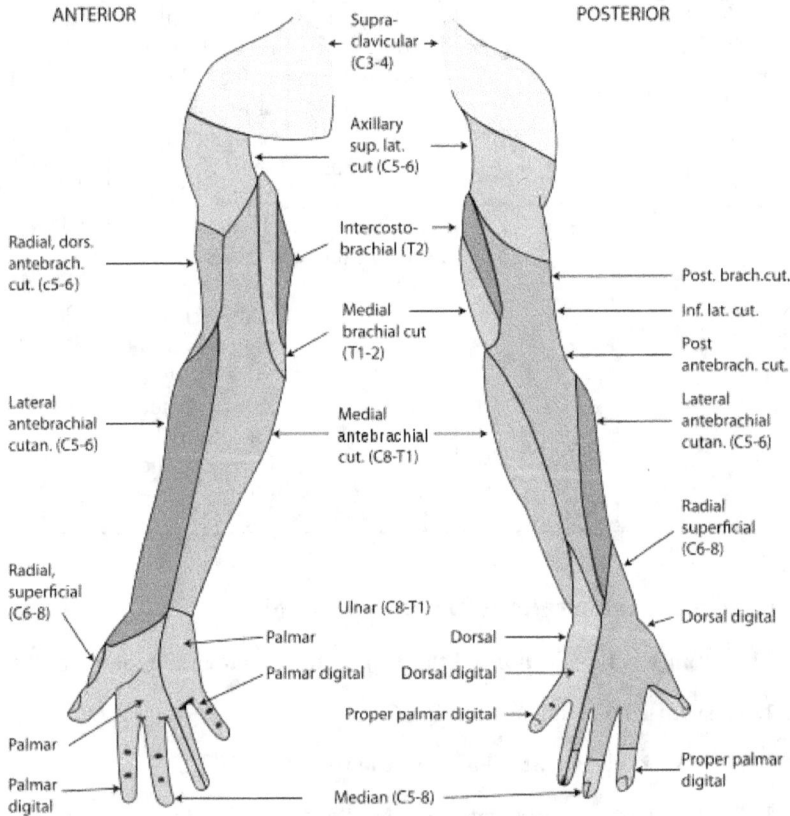

Figure: Cutaneous nerves of the upper limb (Wikipedia.org; Free Encyclopedia)

Notes:

The supraclavicular nerves are derived from the cervical plexus.

The intercostobrachial nerve is derived from the T2.

The upper and lateral cutaneous branches of the arm are branches of the posterior division of the axillary nerve.

The lower lateral cutaneous branch of the arm and the posterior cutaneous nerve of the arm are branches of the radial nerve.

The medial antebrachial cutaneous nerve is a continuation of the musculocutaneous nerve and it begins 2-3 cm above the elbow joint

All the cutaneous branches of the upper limb are derived from the brachial plexus and its branches **except** the supraclavicular nerves and the intercostobrachial nerve.

The medial cutaneous nerve of the forearm and the medial cutaneous nerve of the arm are derived from the medial cord of the brachial plexus.

The cutaneous nerves carry the postganglionic sympathetic fibers to the a. sweat glands b. blood vessels in the dermis and the c. arrector pilorum muscles of the hair follicle. Hence the effects of the sympathetic on the skin are sudomotor, vasomotor, and pilomotor respectively.

An area of the skin innervated by an individual spinal cord segment is called a **dermatome**.

Antebrachial means forearm.

Sudomotor means stimulating the sweat glands

Pain that arises in muscles, tendons, ligaments, and bones is most likely detected by the free nerve endings in connective tissue. This nociceptive endings react to physical trauma and to local chemical alterations, such as those that may be caused by the ischemia.

Sensory receptors are located within and around the capsule of the synovial joints

1. Ruffini-like cutaneous endings 2. Golgi tendon organs 3. Free nerve endings and 4. Small pacinian corpuscles

The Lymphatic System of the Upper Limb

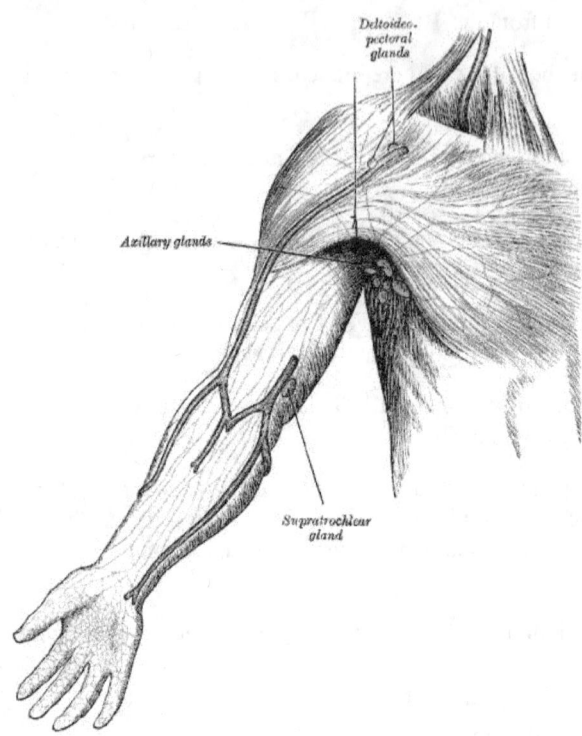

Figure: Lymphatic drasinage of the upper limb (Wikipedia.org; Free Encyclopedia)

The Lymphatic Drainage of the Upper Limb

The lymphatics of the upper limb drain into the **axillary group of lymph nodes.** The superficial lymphatic vessels arise from the lymphatic plexuses in the skin of the fingers, palm, and dorsum of the hand.

The axillary lymph nodes also receive drainage from the upper part of the trunk, the lower neck, the chest, and upper part of the abdominal wall. About 75% of the lymphs from the **breast** drains into the axillary lymph nodes.Changes in axillary lymph nodes may indicate a pathologic process in the breast. The axillary region has about 20-30 lymph nodes.They are arranged into six groupes—1. Humeral (lateral) nodes 2. Pectoral (anterior) nodes 3. Subscapular (posterior) nodes 4. Central nodes 5. Deltopectoral 6. Apical nodes. The lymphatic vessels follow the blood vessels (e.g. cephalic, basillic, and axillary veins) in its **course from fingertips to axilla.**There are a few lymph nodes at the elbow joint called the **epitrochlear or cubital nodes**, which may be enlarged in the **infection of the hand.** The **apical nodes** of the axilla are the most superior groups of nodes in the axilla and drain all other groups of nodes. The efferent lymphatic vessels from the apical nodes form the subclavian lymphatic trunk, these lymphatic vessel drains into the venous system at the junction between the subclavian vein and the internal jugular vein either directly or through the **thoracic duct** in the left side or right lymphatic duct on the right side.

Notes: Breast cancer is one of the most well-known cancers in women. One of the ways of metastatic spread is through the lymphatic vessels that drain laterally into lymph nodes in the axilla and medially into the nodes related to the internal thoracic vessels.

Objective Question

Q. Illustrate the lymphatic drainage of the upper limb.

BIBLIOGRAPHY

1.   Chaurasia's human anatomy. 4th ed. CBS; 2004.

2.   Clinical Anatomy by Regions.Richard S. Snell.8th ed.Lippincott Williams and Wilkins.2007

3.   Cunningham's Manual of Practical Anatomy, G.J Romans, Volume 2;Oxford University Press;1986

4.   Dorland's Pocket Medical Dictionary. 25th ed. Saunders; 1995.

5.   Drake et all, Grays Atlas of Anatomy,2005

6.   Gray's Anatomy for Students Flash Cards. Richard L.Drake, Wayne Vogl and Adam W.M. Mitchhell, Elsevier Churchill Livingstone,2005

7.   Grays Anatomy. 39th ed. Elsevier Churchill Livingstone; 2005.

8.   Grays Anatomy for Students, 1st Edition, Richard L.Drake, Wayne Vogl and Adam W.M. Mitchhell, Elsevier Churchill Livingstone,2005

9.   Langman, Sadler. Medical embryology. 8th ed. Lippincott Williams and Wilkins; 2000.

10.   Grants Dissector, Tank PW . 14th ed. Lippincott Williams and Wilkins; 2008

11.   Metcalf Willium Kenneth. The Anatomy Answer Book. 1st ed. J&B publishers.2006

12.   Moore, KL, Persaud. The developing human: clinically oriented embryology. 7th ed. Philadelphia: Lippincott Williams and Wilkins; 2006

13.   Moore, KL, Dally, AF. Clinically oriented anatomy. 5th ed. Philadelphia: Lippincott Williams and Wilkins; 2006.

.

14.   Halim A. Surface and Radiological Anatomy.2nd edition. CBS Publications, New Delhi. 2007

INDEX

A

abduction 8, 14, 16, 31, 43, 54, 57, 59-60, 95, 137, 144
abductor 41, 104, 109, 115, 131-2
abductor pollicis brevis 115-16, 118, 127
abductor pollicis longus 40, 106-7, 112-13
abducts 55, 99, 105, 109, 131-3, 138
acromial 9-10, 14, 84
acromioclavicu 143
acromioclavicular 1, 4, 6, 8, 17, 59
acromioclavicular dislocation 17
Acromioclavicular Joint 17
acromioclavicular ligament 13
acromion 2, 4-6, 17, 54-5, 59, 65
acromion process 3-5, 9-10, 51-2, 59, 63, 65
acromion process articulates 52
adduction 8, 14-15, 31, 42, 68, 85, 137
adductor pollicis 115, 118, 127, 132, 139
adducts 9, 56, 86, 99, 132-4, 138
anastomoses 33, 62-4, 72-4, 96, 119, 126
anatomical 24, 66, 89, 145
anatomical neck 19, 23-4
anatomical position 3, 10
anatomical snuff box 38, 96, 104, 107, 112, 137, 142, 145
anconeus muscle 29
angeal joints 133
angle 3, 5-6, 25, 47, 53
  superior 8, 53
anterior 5, 15, 19-20, 23-4, 27, 29, 33, 41-3, 55, 61, 65-6, 68, 73, 84-7, 100-1, 104, 109, 120, 132, 142, 144-5, 148
anterior aspect 26-7, 40, 77, 103
anterior border 12, 29, 113
anterior branch 91
anterior compartment 76, 101, 103, 107, 141
anterior cutaneous nerve 142
anterior descending branch 66
Anterior dislocation of shoulder 13
anterior divisions 88
anterior fibers 15
anterior-inferior dislocations 95
anterior interosseous 103
anterior interosseous artery 103, 141
anterior interosseous nerve 103, 108, 113, 142
anterior- posterior radiograph 34
anterior side 114, 120
anterior surface 23, 78, 85, 104, 118-19, 140
anterior ulnar 73
anterior wall 85-6
anterolateral 24
anterolateral surface 23-4

anteromedial 23-4, 142
anteromedial surface 23-4
Anteroposterior radiograph 31-2, 45
aponeurosis 70, 78-80, 85, 99, 132
apular 14-15
ar ligament Anterior 14
arches 9, 41-3, 65, 126, 130
arm 1, 8-10, 18-19, 35, 47, 55-8, 60, 62, 65-7, 69, 71-2, 74-7, 80, 84-7, 91-2, 94-6, 142, 144-7
Arm Muscles 66
armpit 1, 80
artery 14-15, 24, 33-4, 38, 42-3, 61, 63, 65, 72-4, 80, 84, 103-4, 118, 125, 144
  deep 74
  thoracoacromial 84-5, 87
artery Posterior 15
artery Suprascapul 14-15
articular 41, 118, 141
articular branches 77
articular disc 16-17, 39
articulates 10, 19, 25, 30, 39, 65, 118
articulating, joint 14, 33, 41
articulating surfaces 17
ascending branch 23
attachment 12-13, 17, 22-3, 25-6, 29, 65, 113, 124, 130, 137-8
  capsular 24
  palmer interosseoi 115
Attachment of Ligaments 3-4
Attachment of transverse humeral ligament 23
Attachment to Coronoid Process of Ulna 29
Attachments of Clavicle 12
axial line 137
axilla 1, 6, 61-2, 76-7, 80-1, 83-7, 95, 149
Axillary 55-6, 92
axillary artery 62, 64, 72, 81, 83-5, 87-8, 95-6, 103
axillary border 5-6
Axillary border of scapula 2
axillary nerve 24, 26, 28, 57, 61-3, 76, 84-5, 91, 95, 147
  brachial plexus.The 62
axillary nerve injury 63
axillary skin 145
axillary veins 82-3, 95-6, 148

B

ball 7, 15, 139
bands 114
  single median 114
base 8, 17, 39-40, 45, 78-9, 99-101, 105-6, 109, 112, 114, 117, 125-7, 129, 131-2, 138-40

Base of proximal phalanx   45
basilic vein   95-7, 142-3
biceps   7, 24, 33, 71, 80, 90, 93, 142
biceps brachii   3, 22-3, 27, 30, 53, 58, 65-7, 70-2, 76, 80, 84, 93, 96
biceps brachii muscle   7
biceps brachii muscle tests spinal cord segment C5   79
biceps brachii tendon   66, 70-1, 76, 79, 104
biceps brachii tendon b.brachial artery   79
biceps reflex   71, 79-80
bicipital   56, 67, 70, 78-80
bicipital aponeurosis   70, 97
bicipital groove   22-3
bipennate   133-4, 137
blood pressure   72, 79-80
blood supply   38, 40, 126, 140
blood vessels   111, 129, 147-8
bones   1, 9, 11, 13-14, 18, 22, 31, 33, 35, 38-43, 47, 58, 60, 73, 99-100, 105, 107, 109, 112, 132-3, 137, 147
   fractured   16, 38
   funny   77, 107
   long   9, 11, 13, 19, 28, 39
   lunate   38-9
   sesamoid   39-40, 118
   trapezium   39
bones.The distal heads   40
border   4-7, 12, 23-4, 29, 53-7, 72, 80, 84-6, 95, 100, 106
boundaries   61-2, 78, 80, 95, 112
boxer   138
brachial   24, 34, 80, 95, 139, 143-5
brachial artery   28, 35, 65, 70, 72-5, 77, 79-80, 84, 96-7, 103-4
   deep   72, 74
Brachial Nerve Lesions   93
brachial plexus   13, 16, 74, 76-7, 83, 85, 87-92, 95, 101, 103, 107, 142, 147
brachial veins   96
Brachialis   23, 27, 33, 65, 68, 76, 90, 106
brachialis muscles   24, 29, 76
brachii   7, 24, 33, 75, 80, 90, 142
brachii artery, profunda   24, 28, 74-5
brachii muscle   29
   weakness triceps   75
brachii Pronation   33
brachioradialis   23, 26, 75, 79, 91, 93, 106-7, 131, 142
brachioradialis muscle   76, 79, 104, 106
brachioradialis tendon   106, 108, 125
branch/continuation   103
branches   24, 42-3, 62-3, 65, 72, 74, 76-7, 83-4, 88, 90, 92, 95-6, 100, 103-4, 117-18, 125, 131-4, 141, 143-5, 147
   collateral   88
   deep   63, 79, 92, 106-7, 109-10, 118, 127, 132, 134, 137, 141-2
   digital   126-7, 137

independent   142
largest   74
muscular   95, 104
palmer   126
superficial   79, 106, 112, 118, 126, 128, 137, 141-2, 145
brevis   25, 38, 105, 107, 109, 118, 127, 131-2
bridge   60

C

C8   131-2
canal   118
capitate   37-9, 45, 132
capitulum   25-6, 30, 32-4, 40
capsule Medial   43
carpal   39, 41-2
carpal bones   1, 37, 39-40, 42, 120
   displaced   39
   distal row of   40, 43
carpal tunnel   119-21, 126, 140
carpal tunnel syndrome   39, 113, 120-1, 124, 126
Carpometacarp   42
carpometacarpa   42
carpometacarpal   44, 109-10
carpus   38-9, 41
cartilages   14, 85-6
cavity   7-8, 18, 55, 57
   joint   18, 59
centers, primary   11-12
cephalic vein   85, 87, 96-7, 112
children   34-5
   young   35-6
circumduction   14, 42
circumflex   15
circumflex scapular artery   61, 63, 84
circumflex scapular artery disrupts   62
clavicle   1-2, 4, 6, 9-14, 16-18, 47, 52, 54-5, 65, 80, 85-7, 145
   female   10
   fractured   17
   left   11
clavicle articulates   1
clavicle fracture   16, 18
clavicle Sternocostal   85
clavicular   14, 84-5
   pectoral nerve   85
clavicular fracture   13, 16
clavicular head   12, 96
clavicular shaft   10
clavipectoral fascia   13, 84-5, 95-6, 135
CN   54, 57, 87
collateral   33, 41, 43, 73
collateral artery   74, 77
   inferior ulnar   27, 72-3
collateral nerves   91
Colles fracture   36
comm   105-6

compartment syndrome 141
compartments 16, 111-12, 131, 141
concave 9-10, 30
contour, rounded 57, 66
contracture 130, 135, 141
convex 9-10, 25
coracobrachialis 3, 53, 65, 68, 76, 80, 84, 90, 92
Coracoclavicular 8
coracoclavicular ligament 3, 12, 17
coracoclavicular ligament damage 17
coracoid process 2-3, 5, 17, 52-3, 58
coracoids 3, 6, 58, 60, 68, 86
cords 85, 87-91, 130, 139
   lateral 76, 88, 92
coronoid 25, 68, 99-101
coronoid process 26, 28-30, 32, 35, 40, 111
costal 9, 14, 85-6
costal surface 3, 7, 53
Costoclavicu 14
CP Coronoid process of ulna 32
crest 52, 54-5, 109
cubicles 113
cubital 100, 103-4
cubital fossa 65, 72, 78-80, 96-8, 104, 106, 110, 142
cuff 55
cular 14
cutaneous 79, 87, 107, 141, 144-5
Cutaneous branches 146-7
   lateral 147
cutaneous innervations 47, 118, 137, 145
cutaneous nerves 91, 146-7
   lateral 76, 79, 90, 142
   lateral antebrachial 142, 146
   lateral antibrachial 76
   lower lateral 145
   medial antebrachial 142, 146-7
   superior lateral 63
   upper lateral 47, 145
cutaneous sensation 76, 126

D

damage 16, 57, 74-6, 141
Deep branch of radial 105
Deep Flexor Muscles 100, 102
Deep Layer of Muscles 109
Deep muscles 110
deep palmar arch 103, 125, 130, 134
deltoid 15, 47, 52, 55, 58-9, 61, 63, 70, 74, 84, 91, 93, 95
deltoid muscle 4, 12, 22-4, 47, 61, 63, 95
deltoid muscle-Deltoid 58
deltoid muscle forms 57
deltoid tuberosity 23-4, 55, 66
Deltopectoral 148
depression 8, 14, 26, 63
   small 26

diaphysis 22, 24, 27, 45
digital arteries 117, 125-6
   common 126
digitations 53
digiti 132
digitorum 41, 100, 106
digits 45, 117-18, 126, 129, 134, 145
disc 16, 30, 41
disc Interclavicul 14
Dislocated lunate 39
dislocation 16-18, 35, 59
distal 25, 30, 37, 39-40, 45-6, 52, 72, 99-101, 109, 112, 114, 116, 118, 127, 140
distal border 126
distal branches 38
distal interphalangeal 139
distal interphalangeal joints 103, 115
distal lesion 142
distal phalanges 114, 126, 140
distal phalanx 45, 109, 114, 138, 140
distal radius 36
Distal Radius and Ulna 36
distal row 39
distribution 121, 141
divisions 88-9, 147
dorsal 6-7, 30, 41-2, 56, 105-6, 115-16, 133
Dorsal aspect of base 109
dorsal interossei 114-15, 118, 121, 136-7, 139
dorsal interossei muscles 104, 137, 139
dorsal scapular 56-7, 90
dorsal scapular nerve 57, 92
dorsal surface 51, 79, 142
dorsal venous network 96, 143
dorsomedial aspect 96
dorsum 75, 79, 107-8, 112-14, 141-2, 145, 148
downwards 16, 53, 62, 65, 77, 103-4, 139
   radius projects 43
drain 149
drainage, lymphatic 148-9

E

eal 106
elbow 1, 24-6, 28-31, 33-5, 65, 68-9, 71-7, 80, 94, 96, 99, 104-5, 107-8, 147-8
   extended 93
   repetitive 108
Elbow Arthritis 35
elbow band 66
elbow dislocations 35
elbow flexion 93
Elbow Joint 31, 34-5
Elbow Joint/Superior Radioulnar Joint/Inferior Radioulnar Joint 32
elbow radiographs 31
elbow region 29, 103, 107
elbow x-ray 34

elevates 54, 56, 86
Elevation 8, 14
Encyclopedia 5-6, 78, 94, 98, 136, 146
entrapment 108, 142-3
  radial sensory nerve 108
epicondyle 25, 27-8, 32, 73-4, 99-101, 105-6, 109, 141
Epiphyseal Lines 22
Erb-Duchenne Paralysis 93
expansio 106
expansion 109, 114-15, 133
  digital 115-16
extension 33, 43, 66, 68-9, 113, 115
extensor 41-2, 94, 105-6, 108-9, 111, 113, 115, 137, 142
extensor carpi 41-2
extensor carpi radialis 25, 107
extensor carpi radialis brevis 113
Extensor carpi radialis longus 25-6, 108, 113
extensor carpi ulnaris 25, 29, 39, 107, 113
Extensor digitorum 25, 107, 113-14
extensor expansion 114
extensor indicis 107, 113, 115
extensor pollicis brevis 106-7, 112
extensor pollicis longus 30, 107, 112-14
extensor retinaculum 106, 112-13
extensor tendons 112, 114, 134-5, 139

F

fascia, deep 66, 70, 76, 78, 85, 96, 104, 112, 129
fibers
  lower 54-5
  sympathetic 144, 147
Fibres 90-1
fibrous 14-15, 114
finger extensors 75
finger prick 140
finger width proximal 126
fingers 1, 40-1, 43, 75-6, 94, 100-1, 106-9, 114-16, 118, 121, 125, 133, 138-41, 148
  baseball 139
  half 91, 142
  little 1, 100, 103, 108, 119, 128, 130, 132, 137-8, 140
  mallet 139
  ring 1, 43, 100, 126, 130, 138, 140
Five bolded nerves 91
Flat shoulder deformity 95
flexed wrists 121
flexes 99-101, 105, 131-3
flexion 14-15, 26, 33, 41-3, 67-8, 73, 76, 80, 85, 103, 113, 115
flexor 29, 41, 91, 99-101, 111, 131-3
flexor carpi 41-2, 99, 118, 130
flexor carpi radialis 25, 131
flexor carpi ulnaris 25, 27, 29, 91, 101, 103-4, 107, 119, 130, 141

flexor digitorum 25, 101, 107, 117, 120, 140
flexor digitorum profundus 29, 101, 103-4, 107, 120, 136, 140-1
flexor digitorum profundus tendon 137
flexor digitorum superficialis 104, 120, 140-1
flexor digitorum superficialis muscle 140
flexor muscles 70, 75
flexor pollicis brevis 116, 127
flexor pollicis longus 103-4, 120, 140
Flexor pollicis longus Attachment of ulnar collateral ligament 29
flexor retinaculum 38, 116, 118-21, 124, 126-7, 129-31, 140
flexor surface 140
flexor tendons 103, 118-19, 125, 133-5
  long 117
  overlying 140
floor 23, 38, 85, 103, 110, 112
forearm 1, 25-6, 28, 30-1, 35, 40, 67-8, 70, 73, 75-9, 90-2, 96, 98-111, 121, 126, 131, 140-2, 146-7
  distal 104, 126
  pronated 93
  right 76
  supinated 25
Forearm Anteriorly 104
formation 63, 93, 95, 143
fossa 32, 55, 86, 100, 143-4
  infraspinous 6, 9, 51-2, 62
fossa.It 103-4
fracture 3, 16, 18, 24, 26-8, 34-5, 38, 40, 63, 74, 95, 138, 142
  muscles.Supracondylar 141
Free Encyclopedia 2, 4, 11, 13, 16, 19-21, 31-2, 34, 36-7, 40, 45-6, 48-51, 54, 64, 67, 69-71, 73, 75, 81-3, 89-90, 93-4, 96-7, 102, 107, 110, 114, 116-17, 120, 122-5, 128-9, 135, 138-9, 143
front 23, 28, 30, 65-6, 73-4, 91, 106, 119
Frozen Shoulder 18
functions 1, 10, 39, 57, 60, 65, 93, 111, 124, 126, 128, 130, 134, 138
fusion 22

G

ganglion 113-14, 118
  dorsal wrist 113-14
glenohumeral 7-8, 18, 65
glenoid 7-8, 55-7
glenoid cavity 4-7, 9
glenoid fossa 7, 19
Golgi tendon organs 147
gravity 8, 16
greater tubercle 2, 22, 47, 56, 58-9
groove 10, 23, 25, 30, 39, 56, 68, 71, 106
  deltopectoral 96
  intertubercular 19, 23

spiral   24, 74
subclavian   12-13
groove Medial   68
guyons   118

H

hamate   37, 39, 45, 99, 118-19, 132
hamate bones   39
Hand and Metacarpal Bones   39
head, deep   111
hook   39, 52, 118-19, 132
HR Head of radius   32
humeral   15, 87, 99-101, 107, 148
  posterior circumflex   74
humeral artery   61-2, 84
  anterior circumflex   23, 61, 84
humeroulnar   31
humerus   1-2, 7, 16, 18-28, 30-5, 47, 54-
6, 58-9, 61-3, 66, 68, 71-5, 78, 85-6, 95,
99-101, 105-7, 109, 111, 141
  lar groove of   86
humerus.The anterior   84

I

inability   57, 60, 75, 121, 144
index   43, 100, 103, 106, 109, 115, 121,
128, 133, 137, 140
index finger   1, 109, 119, 125-6, 138, 140
inferior   3, 5, 33, 47, 52-3, 68, 72, 86, 88
inferior angle   4-7, 53, 56-7, 65, 86
inferior border   55, 61, 74, 84
Inferior dislocation of shoulder   13
inferior surface   11-13, 17, 52
inferior ulnar   74
Inflammation   59, 120, 140
infraspinatus   15, 22, 52, 55, 58, 69, 90,
93, 144
injury   27, 35, 57, 59, 75, 77, 79, 93, 95,
139
  extensor tendon   139
innervations   40, 79, 144
insertion   9, 12-13, 22, 24, 30, 40, 54, 67,
72, 77, 85, 99-100, 105, 109, 131-2, 138,
140
Insertion of anconeus muscle   29
Insertion of brachialis muscle   29
Insertion of pronator teres   104
Insertion of subscapularis muscle   23
Insertion of tendon   70
Insertion of triceps brachii muscle   29
insertion tendons   116
Interclavicular   12
intercostals   144
intercostobrachial nerve   83, 145, 147
Intermediate phalanx of middle finger   45
intermuscular septa, lateral   65-6
intermuscular septum, lateral   26, 66
interosse   41-3

interossei   115, 125, 133, 139
interosseous   29-30, 33, 42, 100-1, 106-7,
109-10
interosseous artery, common   103-4
interosseous borders   1, 29-30, 111
interosseous membrane   1, 30, 103, 111
interosseous nerve   33, 107
interphalangeal   43, 101, 106, 109, 115-
16, 133, 137, 145
interphalangeal joints   44, 94, 128, 137
intertubercu   86
intertubercular sulcus   22-4, 58, 71, 80
ischemia   141, 147

J

joints   1, 8, 14, 17, 41-3, 60, 100, 106-7,
133, 137, 145
junction   13, 16, 86-7, 144, 149

L

lateral aspect   30, 38, 40, 76, 93, 108,
142, 145
lateral border   5-7, 9, 47, 52, 56, 62, 84,
96, 144
Lateral Cord Branches   92
lateral epicondyle   25-6, 32, 34-5, 78, 106
lateral lip   23, 85
Lateral pectoral   90, 92
Lateral pectoral nerve   85
Lateral radiograph   31-2
Lateral root   90, 92
lateral side   26, 79, 96, 115, 125, 142
lateral supracondylar ridges   26, 66
lateral surface   30, 43, 66, 76, 111
lateral thoracic artery   28, 84, 87
latissimus dorsi   8, 15, 23, 57-8, 69, 80,
84, 86, 91
Left scapula   6
lesions   26, 34, 60, 79, 87, 93, 118, 126,
143-4
levator scapulae   53, 92
level   5, 7, 10, 77, 126, 141
life, intrauterine   12, 22
ligaments   3-4, 9, 12-14, 16, 32-3, 35, 41-
3, 57, 59-60, 73, 119, 132, 144, 147
  annular   30, 35
  conoid   12, 17
  coracoacromial   3-4, 59
  costoclavicular   12
  scapholunate   38
  spinoglenoid   9
  trapezoid   12, 17
ligamentum   54, 56
location   95, 112, 115, 117, 130, 137-8
long finger flexors   94
longus   41-2, 99, 101, 105, 107, 109, 125,
129, 145
loss   75-6, 93, 95, 103, 120, 126

loss of cutaneous   79
loss of sensation   75-6, 108
lower border   5, 7, 52, 62, 79, 84, 95-6, 110
lower lateral cutaneous branch   147
lower limbs   1
lower subscapular nerve   57
ls   133
lumbrica   133
lumbrical muscles connect   137
lumbricals   114-15, 121, 125, 133-4, 136-9
  lateral   137
lumbricals flexes   128, 137
lunate   37, 39, 41, 45
lymph nodes   148-9
  axillary   83-4, 87, 148
  deltopectoral axillary   87
lymphatic vessels   87, 148-9

M

Male clavicle   10
manubrium   14, 16
manubrium sterni   9-10
MCQ Q.Which muscles   121
medial   4-7, 9-14, 16, 23-5, 27, 31, 51-3, 56-7, 59, 62, 65-6, 68, 70, 72-3, 77-80, 85-7, 91, 96, 99-101, 103-4, 107, 112-13, 118, 132, 136, 145
  clavicular fracture   17
  fractured   13
medial aspect   30, 130, 132
medial bone   28
medial border   3-6, 24-5, 52-3, 62, 65, 84
medial boundary   100
Medial Cord Branches   92
medial cords   77, 88, 92, 103, 142, 147
medial cubital vein   80
medial cutaneous   79, 91
medial cutaneous nerve   142, 145-7
Medial cutaneous nerve of arm   92
Medial cutaneous nerve of forearm   92
medial direction   111
medial displacement   16
medial edge   79
medial epicondyle   25-7, 32, 34-5, 72-3, 77, 101, 107, 111
medial head   24, 75, 77
Medial head of triceps   24
medial intermuscular septum   66
medial intramuscular septum   77
medial lip   23, 56
Medial lip of intertubercu   86
medial lumbricals   137, 139
medial margin   4, 25, 40, 78
medial margin forms   22
medial pectoral   85, 91-2
medial pectoral nerve   90
medial root   91-2
medial rotation   15

medial side   10, 24, 77, 91, 96, 99, 106, 117, 126, 132
Medial side of palmar   132
medial skin   91, 132
medial supracondylar ridge   25
medial surface   29
medial wall   86
Medially- lunate   38
median   33, 35, 70, 80, 90-1, 97, 99-100, 131-3, 137, 142
median artery   141
median cubital vein   70, 79-80, 96-7
median nerve   26-8, 33-4, 70, 76-7, 79-80, 91-2, 97-8, 100, 103, 111, 113, 116-17, 119-21, 126-7, 130, 138, 140-2, 146
median nerve innervates   116, 127
median nerve supply   127
membrane   100, 107, 109-10
metacarp   105-6
metacarpal bones   39-40, 112, 125, 131-3, 137
  five   1
  third   131
metacarpal bones form   39
  five   39
metacarpals   37, 39-40, 45, 99-100, 103, 109, 112, 114, 132-3, 138
metacarpophal   133
Metacarpophala   43
metacarpophalang   106
metacarpophalangeal   44, 100-1, 109, 115, 130-2, 137
metacarpophalangeal joints   75, 94, 128
middle   1, 10, 13, 16, 23-4, 26, 63, 66, 72, 74-5, 77, 86, 88, 99-100, 106, 109, 111, 114-15, 117, 121, 126, 128, 133, 137-8, 140
middle collateral branch   74
middle fibers   54-5
middle finger   1, 43, 45-6, 103, 115, 121, 137-9
middle phalanx   114, 140
middle shaft   27
middle supraclavicular nerve   11
middle trunks   88, 95
midshaft   27, 68, 74
minimi   107, 115, 132
  extensor digiti   25, 113
Mnemonics   58, 60, 88, 92
mobile   43
Mode of insertion of Flexor Digitorum Superficialis   140
Mode of insertion tendons   116
movements   8, 14, 17, 32, 35, 41-3, 57, 59, 108
Multiple muscular branches   74
muscle Articular   143
Muscle Attachment   11, 52-3
Muscle Attachments on Spine   52
muscle belly   71

muscle fibers 141
muscle Infraspinatus 143
Muscle/Ligament 12
muscle mass 120
muscle spasm 94
muscle tendon 130
muscles 1, 3-4, 6-9, 12-14, 16-17, 22, 24, 27, 32, 35, 40-1, 47, 53-5, 57-60, 63, 65-7, 69, 72, 76, 84-5, 88, 90-1, 93-5, 99-100, 103-5, 107-9, 111, 115-16, 123-4, 130-5, 138, 140-1, 144
  adductor pollicis 104, 125, 134
  arrector pilorum 147
  bipennate 137
  brevis 118
  coracobrachialis 23-4, 76
  deep extensor 40
  digiti minimi 115
  dorsal interosseous 125
  extensor 75, 91
  extensor indicis 114
  flexor carpi radialis 104
  flexor carpi ulnaris 39, 101, 104, 107
  hypothenar 118, 132, 142
  infraspinatus 52
  intercostals 84
  interossei 103, 134, 137
  interosseous 115
  intrinsic 40, 79, 115, 118-19, 131-2, 141-2
  lumbrical 127-8, 138
  major 6, 12, 16, 72, 77, 95-6
  middle scalene 92
  minor 61, 63, 85, 95
  opponens pollicis 40
  palmar interossei 40
  pollicis longus 104
  profundus 101, 107
  rotator cuff 58-9
  scalene anterior 65
  serratus anterior 53, 84
  small 91, 94, 136
  sternocleidomastoid 12, 16
  sternohyoid 12-13
  subclavius 12-13, 87, 90
  supraspinatus 57
  surrounding 61
  trapezius 4, 12, 57, 87
  unipennate 137
  unipinnate 137
muscles form 60
Muscles Innervated 103
muscles pass 130
muscles supinate 40
Muscular Attachments 3-4, 10, 23-5, 40
Musculocutaneous 33, 67-8, 90, 92
musculocutaneous nerve 27-8, 71, 76, 92, 98, 108, 142, 147
musculocutaneous nerve pierces 92

N

Name 5, 9, 14, 32, 35, 40-1, 100, 131-2
Navy 60
neck 9, 23-4, 30, 38, 72, 87-8, 138
Neck of radius 32
nerve 9, 14-15, 26-8, 33, 41-3, 54-7, 67-8, 70, 74-7, 79, 83, 85-7, 90-1, 93, 95, 98-101, 103, 105-10, 114, 118, 129, 131-3, 137, 139, 143-6
nerve Dorsal 42
nerve endings, free 147
nerve fibers 76, 87
nerve innervates 107
  axillary 63
nerve Muscul 15
nerve Posterior 42
nerve results 95
nerve root 90
nerve supply 9, 32, 54, 67, 85, 99, 105, 109, 131-2, 139
Nerve Supply Thenar 131
nerve Suprasc 15
ngeal joints 43
nodes 148-9
  apical 148-9
notch 14, 25, 30, 33, 52
  scapular 143
  spinoglenoid 52
NR Neck of radius 32
numbness 107-8, 121
  ulnar nerve distribution 94
nutrient artery 13, 24
nutrient foramen 13, 24

O

Objective question, suprascapular vessels 13
oblique 38, 134, 138
olecranon 25, 28-9, 32, 68, 77, 100, 105
olecranon bursa 29
olecranon process 26, 28-9, 32, 77
Opponens 131-2
origin 3, 7, 9, 12, 23-4, 26, 29, 39-40, 53-4, 58, 62, 67, 70, 72, 75, 85, 99-100, 105-6, 109, 111-12, 131-2, 136, 143
  common extensor 25, 35
  common flexor 35
  site of 7
Origin of brachioradialis 23
Origin of flexor 29
Origin of flexor digitorum profundus 29
Origin of teres 6
Origins of muscles 7
ossification 11-12, 29
  primary center of 22
ous 15, 41-3
overuse strain 35

P

pain 35, 54, 63, 107-8, 113, 120-1, 141-3, 147
pal 42-3
palm 104, 112, 117, 121, 124-6, 128-9, 132-4, 140-1, 145, 148
palmar 41-3, 99-100, 117-18, 126, 130, 132, 137, 139
  deep 126, 130
Palmar and Dorsal interossei Muscles 137
palmar aponeurosis 117, 129-30, 135
palmar,arch 125-6, 134
palmar branch 117, 126
  deep 125
Palmar branch of median nerve 126
palmar brevis muscle 128
palmar carpal branches 104
palmar interossei 114, 133, 136-7
palmar surface 39, 126, 131
palmaris brevis 118, 130, 135, 137
Palmaris longus 25, 41, 119
Palmaris longus muscle 130
palmer surfaces 39, 121, 137
paralysis 57, 63, 75-6, 94-5
Parona, space of 140
pass
  muscles tendons 130
  suprascapular vessels 60
patient 18, 75, 94, 108, 121, 130
pectoral 14, 16, 84, 148
pectoral girdle 6, 10, 47
pectoral region 1, 14
pectoralis 3, 8, 12, 15-16, 23, 53, 58, 70, 80, 84-5, 87, 90-1, 96, 145
phalanges 1, 39-40, 100, 114, 137
phalanx 40, 114, 131-3
phrenic nerve 144
Physiological Scapulothoracic Joint 8
pierces 77, 92, 96, 107, 144
pisiform 39, 45, 99, 118-19, 132
  muscle.The 39
pisiform bone 118
Pivot 33
plane 42, 44, 76
plexus 88, 95, 139, 143-4
pollicis 41, 101, 109, 131
  opponens 116, 118, 127
posterior 6, 14, 19, 21, 29, 33, 41-3, 54-6, 61, 65, 67-8, 73-4, 77, 80, 86-7, 91, 100, 105-7, 109, 142, 147-8
posterior aspect 3, 26-7, 62, 74
Posterior Attachment 24
posterior border 6, 12, 28-9, 52
posterior branches 74, 91, 104, 142
posterior circumflex 61-2, 84
posterior circumflex humeral artery 24, 61, 63, 84
posterior compartment 66, 74-5, 107, 141
posterior cord 62, 74, 88

Posterior Cord Branches 92
posterior cutaneous nerve 146-7
posterior divisions 88
posterior fibers, biceps brachii Extension 15
posterior humeral circumflex artery 28
posterior interosseous 79, 107
posterior interosseous arteries 104, 107
posterior interosseous nerve 107-8, 110, 113, 141-2
posterior interosseous nerve innervates 107
posterior scapular regin 59
posterior scapular region 62-3
posterior surface 13, 24, 26, 56-7, 107, 112
posterior ulnar recurrent 72
posterior wall 62, 84, 86
posteromedial 144
postganglionic 144, 147
pressure 70, 75, 80, 107-8, 119, 141
process 3-6, 28-9, 52, 54, 56, 58-60, 68, 86, 99-101, 105, 108
profunda brachii 74
  arteria 72, 74
profunda brachii vessels 62
profundus 100, 117, 120, 140
Pronates 99, 101
pronation 70, 105
Pronator 33, 99, 101
pronator quadratus 103-4
pronator teres 25, 29, 77-8, 100, 104, 111
pronator teres forms 100
pronator teres muscle 104, 111
protraction 8, 14
proximal 16, 22-3, 28, 37, 39-40, 43, 46, 77, 100, 108-9, 114, 126, 131-3
proximal bases 39
proximal interphalangeal joints 103, 130
proximal phalanges 40, 115, 140
proximal phalanx 45, 109, 114, 139-40
proximal row 37, 39
Pulled elbow/Nursemaid's Elbow 35

Q

quadratus 33, 101

R

radial 24, 33, 38-9, 41, 67-8, 72-4, 79, 91-2, 105, 108-10, 112, 119, 126, 138
radial artery 38, 72, 96, 103-4, 106, 111-12, 117, 119, 125-6, 131, 134
radial bursa 140
radial collateral arteries 74, 79
radial collateral ligament 26, 31
radial groove 24, 26, 74-5

radial nerve   24, 26-8, 33, 62, 66, 68, 74-6, 79, 91, 98, 106-8, 110, 112, 125, 137, 141-2, 145-7
  superficial   107-8
Radial Nerve and Posterior Interosseous Nerve   141
radial nerve innervates   107, 141-2
radial nerve results   79
radial notch   28, 30
Radial Notch of Ulna   30
Radial origin of flexor digitorum superficialis 104
Radial origin of flexor pollicis longus   104
radial recurrent artery   74, 104
radial styloid process   30, 45
radial tuberosity   30, 32, 70
radialis, carpi   41, 105
radioulnar   33
  superior   30-1
radius   1, 25-6, 28, 30-6, 38-40, 43, 45-6, 72, 99-101, 104-5, 107, 109, 111, 113, 142
radius Branches   104
radius distal   109
radius Radial notch   33
Radius Scaphoid   41
Recurrent   131
recurrent artery, anterior ulnar   73
recurrent branch   116-17, 126-7, 131
regain muscle usage   93
Relations of Pronator Teres Muscle   111
resistance   57-8, 94, 106, 134
retinaculum   99, 119, 131-2
retraction   8, 14, 57
rhomboids   8, 52-3, 56-7, 90, 92
Rib Levels   5
ribs   2, 5, 14, 16, 56, 65, 80, 84-6, 95
ridge   10, 99, 105
roof   78-9, 97, 112
roots   17, 51-4, 56, 60, 88-90, 93-4, 144
rotation   8, 57, 85-6, 95
  lateral   15-16, 59, 93
rotator   55
rotator cuff   18, 59-60
rotator cuff syndrome   59
rupture   71

S

saddle   14, 42, 44
scaphoid   37-40, 45, 112, 119, 131
scaphoid bone   38-9
scapula   1-10, 17-19, 40, 47, 51-60, 63-5, 67-9, 80, 85-6, 94-5, 143-4
  levator   8, 57
  opposite   94
  winged   94
scapula Muscles   58
scapulae   16-17, 56, 90
scapular   2, 144
scapular ligaments   9, 60

  variable inferior transverse   9
scapular region   1, 47, 54
scapulothoracic   8
secondary ossification centers   34
sensation   75-6, 95, 108, 142
sensory   54, 107-8, 118, 144
sensory nerve   79
septa   66
serratus   86, 144
Serratus anterior   8-9, 70, 80, 84, 90
Sex differences of clavicle   10
shaft   1, 10, 12, 19, 23-4, 26-30, 39-40, 45, 62, 74-5, 100-1, 104, 111, 132
shoulder   1-2, 8-9, 13, 15-19, 24, 47, 55-7, 59-60, 63, 65-8, 80, 84-5, 93-5, 143-4
shoulder abduction   93
Shoulder and Scapular Region   47
shoulder blade   65
shoulder dislocations   2, 57
shoulder droop   17
shoulder girdle   10, 47
  bones form   50
shoulder pain   71
shoulder region   1, 47
shoulder separation   17
Shoulder X-Ray   2
site   16, 22, 36, 107
skin   4, 47, 60, 63, 75-6, 78, 80, 87, 91-2, 95, 104, 112, 126, 128-30, 142, 145, 147-8
snuff box   145
space, quadrangular   61-2, 84
spinal   54, 56
spinal accessory nerve   57
spinal nerves   88, 95
spine   3-5, 9, 47, 51-7, 65, 87, 144
  scapular   51
Spine of scapula   6
stability   16-17
sternal   9-10, 14
sternoclavic   14
sternoclavicular   1, 12, 16-17, 87
sternoclavicular joints   17
sternum   16-18, 85
stethoscope bell   72, 79-80
styloid process   28-30, 39, 43, 106, 112-13
subacromial bursa   18, 22, 59-60
subclavian artery   13, 64-5, 84, 95
subclavian nerve   87
subclavius   80, 85-7, 90, 95, 144
subclavius muscle acts   87
subcutaneous   4-5, 9, 28-9, 51
subscapular   55-6, 84, 86, 92, 148
  ar artery   15
  lower   9, 91-2
  upper   91-2
subscapular artery   61, 63, 84, 103
subscapular fossa   5, 7, 9
subscapularis   7, 9, 15, 55, 58, 61, 80, 86, 91
subscapularis bursa   18

subscapularis muscle 23
subscapularis.Testing abduction 59
sudomotor 147
Superficial flexor muscle 25, 98-9, 102
Superficial layer of muscles 105
superficial palmar arch 117, 125-6
Superficial palmar branch 104, 125
superior transverse scapular 60
superior transverse scapular ligament bridges 60
superior transverse scapular notch 52
superior ulnar 73, 77
superior ulnar collateral artery 27, 66, 72-3, 103
superoposterior surface 29
supination 33, 67, 70, 76, 105, 111
supinator 27, 33, 75, 78-9, 91, 104, 107-10
supinator muscle 110, 141-2
supinator muscle forms 110
supplies 14, 32, 38, 41, 73-4, 84, 100, 126, 132, 141, 145
supplies articular branches 77
Supraclavicular 145
supraclavicular nerves 47, 145, 147
supracondylar fracture 26, 34-5, 141
supraglenoid tubercle 7, 40, 52, 58, 71
suprascapular 55, 60, 63, 95, 143-4
suprascapular artery 13, 52, 60-2
suprascapular foramen 60
suprascapular nerve 9, 60, 90, 143
suprascapular nerve pass 52
suprascapular notch 5, 17, 60
Suprascapular Notch and Superior Transverse Scapular 60
supraspinatus 15, 22, 52, 55, 58-9, 69, 90, 93, 143-4
supraspinatus tendinitis 59-60
supraspinatus tendon 59
  damaged 59
supraspinous 52, 55, 57
supraspinous fossa 6, 51-2
Surascapula 14
surface 5-6, 9, 14-15, 17, 23-4, 33, 55-6, 65-6, 68, 80, 85-6, 99-101, 105, 109, 132
Surface Landmarks 65-6
surgical neck 23-4, 26, 61-3, 84, 95
sweat glands 147
symptoms 94, 108, 121
syndrome 108, 120-1
  cubital tunnel 107-8
  radial tunnel 108
synovial 4, 14, 30-1, 33, 41-4, 113
  socket type of 7, 15
synovial bursa 60
synovial joints 42, 147
synovial sheath 23, 112, 114, 120, 122, 140-1
  common 140
  digital 140

T

tap 69, 79-80
tendon reflex, deep 71
tendon sheath 113
  common flexor 140
tendons 22-3, 30, 39, 59-60, 69-72, 79-80, 103-4, 106, 112-14, 117-20, 122-4, 129-31, 136, 139-42, 145, 147
  biceps 70
  common 3
  extensor carpi ulnaris 106
  extensor digitorum 139
  flattened 114
  flexor carpi radialis 131
  long 24
  palmaris longus 130
  pisiform bones 113
  pollicis longus 142
  sore 71
teres 6-7, 9, 15, 22-3, 33-4, 56-8, 61-3, 69, 72, 74, 77, 80, 84, 86, 91, 93, 95-6, 99
terminal branches 88, 104, 142
  superficial 146
terminal nerves 91
thenar muscles 118, 120-1, 127, 139, 142
thickest 40
thoracic 5, 14, 54, 86
thoracic nerve, long 28, 83, 90, 144
thoracic spinal nerves 87
thoracodorsal 56, 84, 86, 92, 103
thoracodorsal nerve 57, 91, 103
thoracodorsal nerve innervates 103
thumb 1, 40, 42, 44, 101, 106, 109-10, 112-13, 115-16, 119, 121, 125-6, 130-2, 134, 137, 140-1
  phalanx of 101, 109, 132
thumb Abduction 41
thyrocervical trunk, branch of 63
tingling 107-8, 121
tip 3, 43, 53, 58, 67-8, 139
traction 93-4
transverse cervical artery 63, 65, 92
Transverse head 132, 134
trapezium 37, 39, 45, 112, 119, 131-2
Trapeziums and Serratus anterior 8
trapezius 8, 52, 54, 143
trapezoid 37-9, 45
trauma 108, 141, 143, 147
Traumatic avulsion 93
triangular 24, 37, 41, 46, 129
triangular interval 62-3, 74
triangular space 62-3
tributaries 83, 96
triceps brachii 24, 58, 61-2, 65, 68-9, 75, 91
triceps brachii muscle 7, 29, 75
triceps brachii muscle tests 69
triceps reflex 69

triquetrum   37, 39, 45, 118
trochlea   25-6, 32-3, 40
trochlear   25, 28, 33
trochlear notch   28, 32
trunks   10, 16, 18, 88-90, 95, 148
  lower   88
  upper   93, 143-4
tubercle   38-40, 55, 68, 86, 119, 131
  conoid   12-13
  infraglenoid   5, 7, 58
  lesser   2, 22-3, 55, 58
tuberosity   67-8
type   14, 31-3, 41-4, 140
  medial epicondyle.This   35

U

ular   14
ulna   1, 25-6, 28-34, 36, 39-40, 43, 45-6,
68, 70, 99-101, 105-6, 109, 111, 113
ulna articulates   1
ulna Concave ulnar   33
ulna forms   28
ulna Relations   106
ulnar   30-1, 33, 41-3, 68, 79, 91-2, 96, 99-
100, 118, 132-3, 138
ulnar abduction   35
ulnar arteries   72-3, 79, 100-1, 103-4,
107, 111, 117-19, 125-6
Ulnar Artery Branches   126
ulnar avulsion, associated   36
ulnar bursa   120, 140
ulnar canal   118
ulnar claw   94
ulnar collateral ligament   29, 31, 39
Ulnar collateral ligament of elbow joint   25
Ulnar head   99-101
ulnar heads   107
ulnar nerve   26-8, 33, 35, 39, 66, 77, 79,
91, 98, 101, 103, 107-8, 118-19, 126-8,
130, 134, 137-8, 142, 146
ulnar nerve forms   92
ulnar nerve innervates   101, 107, 118, 128
ulnar nerve posterior   72
ulnar origin   100
ulnar recurrent   104
ulnar recurrent artery   73
ulnar side   39, 112, 128, 138
ulnar styloid process   39, 45
ulnar tuberosity   29
ulnaris   41-2, 99, 118
  carpi   29, 41-2, 106
unbloded nerves   91
undersurface   10, 52, 61
unipennate   133-4
upper border   52, 61-2
upper limb   1-2, 10, 16-18, 35, 40, 64, 71,
87, 92-3, 95, 143, 145-9
upper thoracic nerves   47

V

veins   80, 95-7
  internal jugular   13, 149
venipuncture   97-8
ventral   5, 92, 95, 104
vertebrae   54, 56, 86
vertebral   5-6, 47, 53, 56
vertebral border   3, 5-6, 65, 94
vessels
  circumflex scapular   62
  posterior circumflex humeral   61
vincula   140

W

wall   86, 94
weakness   57, 75-6, 108, 120, 144
weight   1, 17
Wikipedia.org   2, 4-6, 11, 13, 16, 19-21,
31-2, 34, 36-7, 40, 45-6, 48-51, 54, 64, 67,
69-71, 73, 75, 78, 81-3, 89-90, 93-4, 96-8,
102, 107, 110, 114, 116-17, 120, 122-5,
128-9, 135-6, 138-9
winging   94-5, 144
wrist   1, 38-9, 41-5, 75-6, 96, 99-101,
103-6, 108, 112-13, 118-20, 125-6, 130,
134, 141-2, 145
wrist Abducts   105
wrist-flexion test   121

[Created with **TExtract** / www.Texyz.com]